Praise for *Unleash Your Ini*
by Daniele Ha

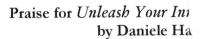

"Daniele's determination to transform her life to what it is today, despite the hardships she has endured, is infectious. She inspires her clients, friends, and the entire diabetes community to live with strength and passion. Anyone will benefit from reading this book."
—**Asha Agar Brown, PWD**
Founder and Executive Director, We Are Diabetes

"Daniele's story of diving headfirst into change with intention and determination is loaded with inspiration. It fills me with hope, courage, and knowledge that I can make positive, lasting changes in my life! You deserve to know Daniele. You need to know Daniele."
—**Scott Johnson, PWD**
Blogger, Patient Advocate, Board Member, Diabetes Hands Foundation

"We become infinitely more powerful when we look at what can be gained from our diabetes rather than what may have been lost. Daniele and her contributors bring this front and center. Here's an opportunity to take back your power."
—**Riva Greenberg, PWD**
Certified Health Coach, Author, *Diabetes Do's & How-To's*

"To paraphrase the late great Yogi Berra, "50% of diabetes is 90% mental." Daniele never lets us forget that we're people first, with diabetes second."
—**Gary Scheiner MS, CDE, PWD**
Owner Integrated Diabetes Services, Author, *Think Like a Pancreas*

"I believe in the power of peer support and sharing our positive stories. Daniele inspires and uplifts all of us through her tireless dedication to share and transform the way we look at diabetes."
—**Christel Marchand Aprigliano, PWD**
CEO of The Diabetes Collective, founder, The Diabetes UnConference

"Daniele has a real, genuine passion for the diabetes community. She has made a visible effort to reach out to other diabetics and constantly strives to make all of our stories known. Together we are stronger, and Daniele exemplifies that perfectly!"
—*Diabetic Danica, RN, PWD*
Popular YouTube Video Blogger

"If you can keep it positive between the ears, the rest is a lot easier to manage. We are not where we want to be yet but we're a long ways from where we were. Taking it a day at the time and knowing Daniele will always be there is priceless...she will always be part of our family."
-*Donna Brannan*
Mother of PWT1D

"Daniele is all about making the best of this life, no matter what health obstacles get in your way -- and she does it with compassion and grace. I send folks her way all the time because I trust that her work is loaded with integrity and love."
Jenni Prokopy
Blogger, Chronic Babe, Author, *Chronic Babe 101*

"Daniele has a passion for helping people see the potential opportunities in the wake of their challenges. From her own compelling personal story, to the way she has risen to become an effective advocate for people with diabetes in the diabetes online community through her engaging interviews and constructive outlook, Daniele proves to the community that those of us who live with chronic disease can be the dynamic change-makers of our own stories."
Melissa Lee, PWD
Patient Advocate and Interim Executive Director, Diabetes Hands Foundation

"Having lived with Type 1 diabetes for 27 years myself, as well as being an RD, CDE professionally, I know how important contact with others who "walk the walk" can be to healthy management. Daniele is a fantastic, positive light in the Diabetes Community. We need more people like her to show how to truly "live" despite the 24/7 nature of life with diabetes."
Jennifer C. Smith RD, CDE, PWD
Director of Lifestyle and Nutrition, Integrated Diabetes Services

"Daniele owns her D! She's what Sugar Surfing is all about: the empowered person with diabetes capable of making the tough choices, learning from the results, then taking control to a new level. Let her show you a new path to living well with diabetes. Her book is a must read"
Stephen Ponder MD, CDE, PWD
Author, *Sugar Surfing,* Medical Director, Texas Lions Camp for Children with Diabetes

"The ultimate key to living well with diabetes lies in one's attitude. It may sometimes feel like a burden, but Daniele's energy, enthusiasm and positive attitude will help those who are struggling to acknowledge the challenges, then move on and actively and successfully manage their diabetes. The online community needs role models - Daniele is a great one to follow!"
Lis Warren, PWD
PWT1D, 50 year Diabetes UK & Joslin Medallist

"Every person – and every family – is made up of a tremendous number of moving parts. T1 is just one of those parts, but a part that requires a lot of informed management every single day. Do it. Then...Define your potential and go after your dreams. Join Daniele Hargenrader, and unleash your Diabetes Dominator!"
Laura Billetdeaux
VP Education and Programs at Children with Diabetes, Founder, Friends for Life Conferences

Unleash Your Inner Diabetes Dominator

How to Use Your Powers of Choice, Self-Love, and Community to Completely Change Your Relationship with Diabetes for the Better

DANIELE HARGENRADER

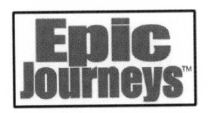

Philadelphia | San Diego

Disclaimer – I am NOT a medical doctor. All information in this book is provided as an informational resource only. It is not to be used for any diagnostic or treatment purposes. This information should not be used as a substitute for professional medical diagnosis and treatment.

Please consult your healthcare provider before making any decisions or changes to your healthcare regimen, and for guidance about the treatment of any specific medical condition. The author and all affiliates expressly disclaim responsibility, and shall have no liability for any damages, loss, or injury whatsoever suffered as a result of the reliance on the information contained in this book as medical treatment. The author is not a medical doctor, and you should always consult with your doctor before changing your healthcare regimen in any way.

Diabetes Dominator and Epic Journeys are a trademark of Epic Journeys Entertainment, LLC

Cover Photography by Rachel Amelio

Cover Design by Bill Hargenrader

Published by Epic Journeys Entertainment
PO Box 14596 | Philadelphia, PA 19115

ISBN: 0692562117
ISBN-13: 978-0692562116

DEDICATION

Dedicated to the superhero inside all of us. It may be lying dormant. It is time to wake it up.

Dedicated to chasing our dreams with wild abandon, and to serving our fellow humans at the highest level possible.

And to my perfect partner Bill. Without your support and belief in my vision, this book would not have been possible. There are no words that can adequately express my love for you.

CONTENTS

FOREWORD – A MOTHER'S PERSPECTIVE

I'm immensely proud to be Daniele Hargenrader's mother. Her passion for life, for optimum health and for helping others to achieve it brings me great joy every day. I wish I possessed even a fraction of her strength and discipline, but having her as a role model inspires me to always strive to do better.

Reading her revealing story in this book has been an emotional roller coaster for me. Years ago when I first learned of her overwhelming depression and binge eating during her teenage years, I searched my brain to try to comprehend how I didn't see how badly she was suffering at the time. If I were reading this book as an objective outsider, I would probably think "what kind of a mother would let her daughter go through all of this pain without getting her help?" But Daniele was very good at hiding it from me because she didn't want to burden me.

So when she acted out and shut me out, I attributed it to regular old teenage angst. I did try to get her to go for counseling when her father died, but she adamantly refused. Many times I suggested diabetes camp; she was having no parts of that. Even as a child, she was always very strong and independent, and as an easy going person who prefers to avoid conflict, I often (usually) let her have her way.

Throughout all of her challenges, Daniele was always a good kid – she never got in trouble; she was always a straight A student and had good friends. Although she never wanted to exercise as a young teen (I couldn't even get her to take a walk around the block!), she did step up to become the manager of her high school boys' soccer team since her boyfriend was the captain!

Something that is probably difficult for younger readers to understand is the lack of information and support that we had about diabetes. We had no computer yet; the internet was in the earliest stages of development and it was years down the road before its widespread use. After her initial diagnosis and a week in the hospital learning the very basic necessities of care such as how to test blood sugars and give insulin injections, we were sent home with a woefully inadequate pamphlet of information. The doctor just told us to test her blood sugar 3 times a day and give insulin twice a day in the amount prescribed, and that was it! We were told that a cure was in the works; it wouldn't be long, maybe a few years away. Still waiting for that, 25 years later. So we learned by trial and error (lots of errors), by reading books and articles, and occasionally advice from very few people who knew something about diabetes. Mostly we figured things out as we went along.

To me, giving Daniele her insulin injections was traumatic – I was very nervous about it and did it slow and hurt her every time, although she claims to have no recollection of it! Fortunately, her father was good at it; he was able to do it quick and easy. But I know she dreaded getting her shot when he wasn't home. We were told in the hospital that children with diabetes normally start self-injecting at around age 12, but our precocious daughter started giving herself her own shots within 3 months of being diagnosed, at age 9! She never wanted anyone to do it for her after that, and that was such a relief for me. From the very beginning, Daniele always wanted to do as much as possible for herself.

Another thing we learned the hard way was how low blood sugars can cause seizures. When I first read information that mentioned that possibility, I didn't think much of it since it had never happened to us, and I assumed it was a rare occurrence. But when it happened the first time at age 14, and I found Daniele writhing on the floor with her eyes rolling back in her head after falling out of bed, we entered a whole new era of worry, fear, and comprehension of the life threatening severity of this disease. The result was many years of a regimen of setting alarms to wake up in the middle of the night to check her blood sugar to avoid lows while sleeping. But just like with every other obstacle, we worked out our best strategies and were always able to cope well and find ways to thoroughly enjoy life despite our challenges! I know it would have made a world of difference for us if only we had an expert guide like this book at that time!

Education is the solution to so many of the problems that plague people with diabetes. Education is also important for others who don't have diabetes; my experience has shown that most people who are not familiar with diabetes think of it as a fairly benign condition – thinking that you just take your insulin and don't eat sugar and go about your business. I'm not referring to traditional academic education, but to down to earth, real life advice that can be implemented immediately, thoughtful recommendations that will bring positive and meaningful results. My fervent hope for this book is that besides providing valuable and practical information for people with diabetes and those who love them, it also brings a revealing personal account of some of the challenges that we face on a daily basis and how they can absolutely be overcome.

Those challenges are different for every person, but we can all relate to the difficulties and discouragement that they can bring. I believe that Daniele's story has the very real potential to increase understanding and compassion. And her amazing transformation and her happiness and success should be a great inspiration to demonstrate that a healthy and joyful life is within reach; it does take effort and determination, but it is possible, rewarding, and extremely gratifying.

I want to let you know that despite all of the trials and tribulations that we went through, we had even more good times, lots of laughter, learning and solving problems together, cooking together, traveling together, and always being there for each other. Daniele is my best friend and greatest inspiration, and I sincerely believe that through this book she will inspire and motivate countless others to take control of their choices, live with passion, gain confidence and robust health, and enjoy an outstanding life!

Gayle Shapiro
Board of Advisors, True You Solutions

FOREWORD – A DOCTOR WITH DIABETES' PERSPECTIVE

Diabetes can be a devastating disease. The rigorous daily demands of constant blood sugar monitoring, multiple insulin injections, mental calculations to determine the correct insulin dose, dealing with high and low blood sugars, plus the lingering fear of complications in the future…it's enough for many to throw up their hands in defeat.

But not Daniele Hargenrader. Type 1 diabetic herself for 24 years, Daniele is an amazing woman who is a powerhouse of information and a much needed source of inspiration for the diabetes community.

I was lucky enough to meet Daniele at The Diabetes UnConference in Las Vegas, in March of 2015. We had met virtually over Google Hangouts just a month or two prior when she interviewed me for her YouTube interview series. During our call, we immediately clicked. I told her about the upcoming conference in Vegas and encouraged her to come and that she could room with me. She got back to me less than a week later to tell me she'd booked her ticket.

My plane arrived around dinnertime but she didn't get in until midnight. I told her that I sleep like a rock so to just come on in whenever she arrived and make herself at home. So we met for the first time in person the next morning when we woke up. We couldn't stop talking for hours, and felt like sisters who had never met. I immediately fell in love with her.

She is one of those vibrant women who radiate positive and genuine energy, lifting the spirits of all fortunate enough to be around her. If and when you meet her, I promise you'll feel better just by being around her motivating and giving spirit.

Diabetes can get you down. I know because I've had it myself for 35 years, since I was 7. It takes a level of responsibility and maturity which is hard to grasp by people who are not affected by this condition. The freedom to enjoy food without any concern is not a luxury for anyone living with diabetes. Every single bite of food must be considered and monitored.

Keeping one's blood sugar in a normal healthy range on a daily basis is essential for enjoying a long and healthy life, yet is not something that is easily achieved by simply taking medication on a daily basis. An endless amount of calculations and considerations must be made hundreds of times every day.

Here are just a sample of thoughts that go through my head on a daily basis to manage my condition, from the second I wake up, until the minute I fall asleep: 'I wonder if I should start my day with a shot of insulin to cover my potentially increased blood sugar due to unpredictable morning hormones? What is a healthy choice for breakfast? How many carbs are in that yogurt? How active will I be today and do I need to adjust my long-acting insulin dose? When and how will I exercise? How will I avoid my blood sugar from going dangerously low? If I go out to lunch, what food choices will be available? How much insulin do I need for that sandwich…will it digest quickly or slowly? Thus should I take a full dose all at once or take two shots a few hours apart? If I go low at any time, do I have a fast-acting sugar source with me? How will my blood sugar stay normal if I have to unexpectedly be active when I was expecting to be sedentary? Or vice versa? If I eat a late dinner, how will I make sure my blood sugar doesn't go dangerously high while I sleep? Or dangerously low, potentially dropping me into a coma, or worse, death? Perhaps I should set my alarm to wake me up at midnight to check…'

Truly, these are thoughts that go through my head, and Daniele's, and those of millions of other people living with diabetes every single day.

I am deeply grateful for having been born with such a driven and tenacious personality, because I fear for people who live with diabetes and yet do not feel they have what it takes to keep up with the daily demands of living with this life-or-death condition.

Living a healthy life with diabetes takes immense focus and determination every single day. If proper care is ignored, consequences are devastating. Diabetic retinopathy is the leading cause of blindness in America. 44% of patients in America with kidney disease have diabetes. In 2010, 73,000 lower-limb amputations were performed on adults with poorly controlled diabetes. It is estimated that 1 in 20 patients with Type 1 Diabetes will experience 'Dead in Bed' syndrome, due to a drop in blood sugar during the night. 65% of people with poorly controlled diabetes die from heart disease and stroke. Adults with poorly controlled diabetes are two to four times more likely to have heart disease or suffer a stroke than people without diabetes. Poorly controlled diabetes is one of the leading causes of death in America.

If you read the headlines, you'd think diabetes is a death sentence. If someone gives in to believing this and just eats what the rest of America is eating, ignores exercise, and has a pity or victim mindset, that is the true recipe for death. Not diabetes itself.

Daniele is absolute proof of that.

She had her days of depression and defeat, like many of us living with diabetes experience. But she found the inner strength and sought out the knowledge to go from being obese to now being the picture of perfect health. With her Omnipod insulin pump on one side of her back and her continuous glucose monitor on the other, Daniele doesn't let diabetes stop her from having an awesome, vibrant, and healthy life.

Her message is truly life-changing and needs to be heard by every person living with diabetes around the globe. In this transformative book, you'll learn all the valuable wisdom she gained along her path from obesity to thriving. She covers the 6 Pillars of Health of The Diabetes Dominator Mentality, which I like to call essential 'prescriptions' for living a healthy life with diabetes.

1. You'll learn about how having the right mindset is a matter of life or death.
2. You'll learn about nutrition, how and what to eat.
3. You'll be reminded how and why exercise is one of your best friends.
4. You'll realize how having a supportive community is some of the best medicine you could have.
5. You'll gain a better understanding of how to take care of your entire body.
6. You'll learn what mindfulness is and how it will benefit your life.

Diabetes can be a death sentence, or it can be a great source of strength. If every single person living with diabetes could read this book and apply Daniele's life-changing wisdom, millions of lives would be improved, billions of dollars would be saved, and the face of health in America would be entirely transformed.

Dr. Jody Stanislaw
Naturopathic Doctor
Living with Type 1 since 1980…and thriving!

AUTHOR'S NOTE

This book is all about taking action. You can get some benefit from this book just by reading it. But you will see an exponentially larger positive impact in your life if you take action when you see the "ACTION ITEM" sections.

It is highly recommended that you keep a journal to track your thoughts and actions as you read through the book. You'll thank yourself in 30 days, or ten years from now when you look back on how much your relationship with diabetes has changed for the better! Your journal can be a document you keep on your laptop, an email you send yourself, a simple spiral notebook, or a leather bound journal.

If you're not ready to keep a journal, then simply take the time to think through the "ACTION ITEM" exercises.

Also, be sure to check out the free accompanying resources and worksheets at diabetesdominator.com/bookresources

To take your experience to the next level, be sure to check out the free accompanying resources and worksheets at diabetesdominator.com/bookresources

Join our supportive community on Facebook: facebook.com/diabetesdominator

Get daily inspiration and motivation on Twitter: twitter.com/diabetesdomin8r

Daniele Hargenrader

INTRODUCTION

The subtitle of this book is: How to use your powers of choice, self-love, and community to completely change your relationship with diabetes for the better. That is a bold statement. But what does it mean? To me it means that instead of diabetes being perceived as a weakness or a curse, that diabetes can actually be a great source of strength if we choose to let it. We all have the power to turn adversity into advantage. Diabetes can be a catalyst for improving our lives, paying closer attention to what matters most in life, and for stepping up and reaching out to be of service to others. I didn't always feel this way, and that's why I wrote this book. This is the book I wish I had when I was younger. This is the book I wish my mom and dad had when times looked darkest.

When I was 9 years old, I was diagnosed with type 1 diabetes. The internet was just a blossoming idea at the time, and my parents were scared out of their minds! There was no Google! We didn't have this invaluable, endless network of information and community at our fingertips that we are so lucky to have available to us today. Diabetes Dominator is much more than a catchy book title or web page. Diabetes Dominator is an identity, a mindset, a superhero mentality that, through incredible losses, struggles, and triumphs, I have created and embodied over the course of the past 24 years. Being a Diabetes Dominator is, more than anything, a mindset. It is a way of life that allows the person who adopts it to be free. It allows us to find liberation from the perceived constraints of diabetes through domination of our fears, limiting beliefs, and inaction. Through many trials and tribulations, great successes and horrible scares, after years of constant frustration, as well as severe mental, emotional, and physical struggles, my Diabetes Dominator was forged.

Diabetes Dominator is an identity and mentality that can be (and is encouraged to be) adopted by anyone who so CHOOSES to step up and be accountable, any person who takes responsibility for their actions and does not place blame for current situations or circumstances on another person, thing, or event. We all share this burden that we call diabetes, no matter what type we have, and nobody wants to be blamed for a 24/7/365 burden that we certainly didn't ask for. However, even though there is no blame that can logically be placed, it is still our personal responsibility to care for our diabetes and to understand, accept, and embrace that it is part of our journey in this life. And maybe eventually, we can come to feel that diabetes didn't happen TO us, but rather FOR us, to help shape us into the incredibly strong, resilient superheroes that each and every one of us is, just for living with the intricacies of diabetes every day.

Having dedicated my life and my studies to nutrition, anatomy & physiology, psychology, and specifically how mindset, food, and exercise affect the human body while living with diabetes, I have strived to become an expert on the subject of diabetes, specifically the aspects regarding its optimal management. I have a Bachelor's of Science degree in Nutrition Science, am a Certified Personal Trainer, a nutritionist, have worked as a personal chef, and have gone through over 500 hours of human psychology training and developed my career through diabetes coaching.

I have had type 1 diabetes for over 24 years, and like many of us, I've been through three stages of life with the disease so far, including childhood, adolescence, and adulthood. I have struggled with incredible loss, severe depression, and an eating disorder, and have come out on the other side, taking myself (with much help from friends, family, and mentors) from what I call "obese to athlete." I have been blessed to find my life's passion and purpose in helping others living with diabetes to embrace their personal power, to step into their Diabetes Dominator mentalities. In my opinion, learning, growing, and contributing never stop if you desire a fulfilling life, and because of this, I have done and will always continue to do research, take classes, and attend seminars and conferences on many topics, including diabetes, nutrition, cooking, exercise science, psychology, and anatomy & physiology.

I've done volunteer work with the American Diabetes Association, including speaking at various YMCA's and Boys' & Girls' clubs, and presented at Camp Freedom, a camp for children with diabetes. I have also had the honor of working with the Children's Hospital of Philadelphia, which has earned the No. 1 spot on U.S. News & World Report's 2013-14 Honor Roll of the Nation's Best Children's Hospitals, where I was lucky enough to speak to recently diagnosed children and their parents about how to live a healthy lifestyle and thrive with diabetes through nutrition and exercise choices, as well as how to cope with the inevitable whirlwind of emotional learning processes required when newly-diagnosed. I have been quoted in Diabetes Forecast Magazine, and my *YouTube* interview series, "Unleash Your Inner Diabetes Dominator," and accompanying blogs have been syndicated on DiabetesDaily. I've written articles for DiabetesMine, Insulin Nation, and Natural Awakenings Magazine, I've been featured in the Philadelphia Inquirer, and have presented at various Fortune-100 companies, teaching people how to live the life they imagined through optimal health.

I genuinely hope that through reading my book, blogs, watching my videos, or interacting with other people with diabetes, that the Diabetes Dominator mentality has the ability to add value to your life, as it has done to mine. I strive to impact the diabetes community in a positive way, and assist people who live with diabetes in implementing changes that will vastly improve the overall quality of their day-to-day lives. It is my vision that the countless people who continue to be transformed through choosing to live as Diabetes Dominators will pass on that excitement, empowerment, confidence, information, and overall value to others through their optimistic, energetic, healthy lifestyles, so that together, we can create an impact on the overall health and outlook of future generations by using a concept as simple and proven to work as leading by example.

We are a community of 387 million people with diabetes worldwide, and the impact that we can have on our community and future generations when we stick together and are focused on any outcome is immeasurable and never-ending. I just want to be a part of our movement as a community to thrive, and to help educate people with diabetes and without diabetes alike to understand that diabetes is far from a condemnation to an impaired life and/or an early death. I want to help make it crystal clear that we can all do and be whatever we want, chase our dreams and passions, and that diabetes can even be a source of incredible power, confidence, and strength if we choose to let it.

This is the book that I wish I could go back and give to my younger self, to tell myself that it's going to be okay. To show myself that there is light at the end of the tunnel, and that instead of feeling weak, hopeless, defeated, and unworthy for the rest of my life, that instead I will end up being stronger than I ever imagined possible.

Since I can't go back and tell myself that, the next best thing I can do now is tell you that. Diabetes can and will make you stronger if you CHOOSE to take the right actions, and believe that you deserve to feel strong, and that you deserve to feel loved.

And if you're beyond that point of feeling that diabetes is a curse, then my hope is that this book will serve as a guide for you to take your life to the next level and give back to the community that needs your voice, your strength, and your light.

"Our deepest fear is not that we are inadequate. Our deepest fear is that we are powerful beyond measure."

Marianne Williamson

PART ONE - YOUR FOUNDATION: DISCOVERING THE DIABETES DOMINATOR MENTALITY

1

THE PROMISE AND BENEFIT OF THE DIABETES DOMINATOR LIFESTYLE

"Don't be discouraged by your incapacity to dispel darkness from the world. Light your little candle and step forward."
-Amma

More people are going to passively sit back and succumb to the complications of poorly controlled blood sugars in the next few years than ever before. Your job is NOT to be one of those people, and my mission is to show you how.

This intro is going to be real. What I am going to tell you is my truth as a person with diabetes for just shy of 25 years, combined with the truths of my clients' experiences. The truth that, for some unfathomable, mind-numbing reason, most doctors don't even mention when diagnosing a patient with diabetes. The truth regarding all types of diabetes and how it relates to you or the person in your life that you love dearly which has prompted you to pick up this book. The truth that is so simple, but has become incredibly skewed and chaotic over the years.

The American definition of "health" has unfortunately become based on a keep-you-sick-and-provide-the-cure-in-a-pill mental state of our country today, combined with some media outlet's deliverance of (mis)information on nutrition, exercise, and how to live healthy lives. Pair all of that with the general lack of interest and motivation of the human population to take full responsibility for our lives and well-being, and willingness to do our own research and find out what has produced the best results for others in our situation, and it is apparent that the overall vision of what is truly healthy is a little more than just blurred–it is barely recognizable. The truth that can set us free of so many of our old diabetes demons.

My goal is not to create more fear, because there is entirely too much of that in the diabetes community as it is, but to inspire the diabetes community to take more directed action that will lead to living our lives feeling empowered, liberated, educated, protected, and confident in our abilities to manage our choices and decisions when it comes to our own diabetes care. More than anything, this is a call to action, a challenge to step up our game of self-love, take things to the next level, and make that next level our new standard. Each of us must become the standard bearers for our own diabetes management. We cannot always have total control over diabetes, this much we all know to be true, but we can control the choices we make with what is available to us regarding our diabetes care, and those choices, in turn, shape our day to day realities.

Every day, we hear on TV, in a magazine or newspaper, online, or from a friend or family member about this amazing new diet program, pill, spray, or some other form of miracle that has been doing wonders for their waistline. That in itself is the first and truly most gargantuan problem of all, one that, if we don't eradicate it from our minds, will almost definitely ensure the failure of any venture into the realm of healthful living. The idea that there is or ever will be any quick fix, magic pill or drink that will make up for the years of damage we have imparted on our bodies (trust me, I spent ten years weighing over 200 pounds with an A1c of 13+%, and I didn't get healthy overnight).

The idea that we can just treat our bodies poorly for any indeterminate amount of time and just take some unregulated supplement to fix the damage we have done in a couple of weeks. The sooner we are able to openly admit that the damage we have done to our bodies, through the lack of attention paid to and priority put on our diabetes care, has taken time, and that the reversal of the damage will also take time, the sooner we will be on our way to healing and recovery, and a resurgence of sustainable energy and confidence that will blow our minds.

I'm not a doctor; however, I can promise you without hesitation that if you choose to begin following the advice laid out in the six pillars of health in this book, the opportunity to see a major difference in the state of your health within four weeks is very real. These changes will come in the form of tighter blood sugar control, lowered doses of insulin or oral meds, fat loss, and increased energy levels, just to name a few. It won't be a miracle, though. It will come as a result of choosing to make different decisions on a consistent basis. One quote that has resonated with me over the years is this: "If you want something you've never had, you must become someone you've never been"- Unknown Author. This is true for any major endeavor that we embark on in our lives, including changing the state of our health.

We must be willing to let go of our old beliefs, habits, and routines, the ones that got us to where we are today. This quote from one of my most influential mentors, Jim Rohn, is along the same lines: "The greatest reward in becoming a millionaire is not the amount of money that you earn. It is the kind of person that you have to become to become a millionaire in the first place." I'm still working on that one, but for now, I can speak to the changes that must be made to change the state of our health. Essentially, we must change who we believe we are and what we believe we are capable of, to some degree, to create sustainable healthy habits. Change is not a bad thing or something to be feared or resisted. Change is truly the only thing that is constant in this world, and our ability and willingness to adapt and roll with the proverbial punches is what shapes our reality day-to-day.

The only thing that will allow our minds and bodies to reshape and restructure themselves, to let go of excess fat and toxins and negative thought patterns, to produce the energy that we desire and deserve every day to make our lives more enjoyable and fulfilling is a healthy lifestyle. A healthy mindset, a healthy nutritional lifestyle, a healthy exercise lifestyle. A lifestyle built around self-love, self-appreciation, choice, community, and action, armed with the knowledge that we are worth it, worth every bit of effort, and we are more than enough for this world. A lifestyle that, without a single word, shows those around us that we are each incredibly valuable, that we all have a purpose in this life, and no passion or dream is too small or seemingly trivial to pursue and share with others if it makes our hearts sing.

A healthy lifestyle is just that, a set of habits and routines that we continually assess, re-assess, shape, and mold to fit our schedules and make us feel proud. A lifestyle that we create and love because it is our own, the choices are ours to make, and that is extremely powerful. It is something that we understand, accept, and embrace as needing to be flexible due, not only to the fact that diabetes care changes with the shape of our days, but also because life is also ever-changing. Therefore, to be successful we must be accepting of and willing to change on a regular basis. One more quote that shapes my way of thinking and that has served me throughout the years is Winston Churchhill's, "Change is the price of survival."

"Anything worth doing is worth doing badly" – G.K. Chesterson. Success is based on taking action using good judgment. Taking action using good judgment is based on experience. Experience is gained through bad judgment or failure and the willingness to learn lessons in those moments of failure. All too often, when we fail at something, we just give up, saying something along the lines of "I tried and it didn't work, so it must not be for me" or, "I gave it a go and didn't get the exact results I had in mind, so this must not be the right answer." I can't tell you how many times this was my thought process and attitude before my transition into embracing what I now call the Diabetes Dominator mentality. However, this is almost never the truth. The truth is that if we examined our original approach, refined our steps based on the first "failure" (aka experience), and decided to try again using a new, different idea or perspective, most likely the second try will be much closer to the target we were originally trying to hit.

And the best part is that we can (and must) keep doing this as often as we need to until we get what we're after, and then we can call all of our "failures" "experience" instead, since that is exactly what they are as long as we are willing to seek out the lessons, the seeds of equivalent opportunity. One of the best parts of failing and gaining experience is that we get to share that with others, and they can learn from our mistakes. In my opinion, the best part of this book is that the reader can learn from my failures, and make progress much faster, progress that took me years of failure/experience to figure out and achieve!

Failure is inevitable and valuable; it is how we react to failure that is what matters most. Every failure we have had has led us to exactly where we are now and has contributed to the strength we possess today. Those valuable experiences have led you to picking up this book with the desire to be the best version of yourself that you can be, to change your relationship with diabetes for the better, the desire to unleash your inner Diabetes Dominator.

2

RESULTS: MY CLIENTS' AND MINE— WE CAN DO IT AND SO CAN YOU

"If you love only yourself, you will serve only yourself. And you will have only yourself."
-Stephen Colbert

As much pride as I have in my own mental and physical transformation, the amount of pride that I have regarding the successes of my clients who, through the coaching process, become my close friends and major sources of fulfillment in my life, is incomparable. That is what I live for. That is what lights me up. That is what fills my heart with so much joy that it becomes overwhelming and on many occasions, brings me to tears. The ability to help others first understand, then accept, and finally embrace their own personal power of choice, to see someone else become electrified with the knowledge that they are powerful beyond measure, is what life is about for me. It is my passion, my purpose, and the reason I feel like I never actually "work," because what I do for a living is what makes my heart smile.

I love to hear from readers of my blog or social media sites, or those who watch my *YouTube* videos about their own "before and after" stories, or stories of any kind of inspiration, or feelings of being able to improve their quality of life after implementing any advice they have heard from me. It is the stories of our diabetes community, the stories of struggle and triumph that fuel my fire, not only to continue helping others, but also to hold myself to the highest level of Diabetes Domination and lead by example. Please don't be shy…write me an email! I am convinced that there is no person with diabetes out there who doesn't have the opportunity to benefit from following the advice in this book, which is based on hard evidence that I have had the pleasure of witnessing, time and time again, through my inspiring clients, students, friends, and family members.

I want to highlight some of my clients' successes, as they are the ones who inspire me to continue fighting the good fight day after day. They inspire me to continue leading by example, and they are the fuel that keeps my fire to share my message, and to encourage others to share their messages, burning strong. They are all a part of our diabetes community, just like you and me. Whether we meet online or in person, we are all part of this amazing tribe, and we are always stronger when we stick together.

Shay and Kathy

I started working with Shay when she was just 16 years old. When we first met, her A1c had been between 9-10% for the past four years. Within three months of working together just one day per week, her A1c dropped to 8%, and her last A1c (June, 2015) was 7.0%. She is now 21 years old, a senior in college on her way to becoming a pediatric nurse, and has beautifully stepped into her Diabetes Dominator mentality. She is relentless at trying different things, being willing to change and adapt. Through the struggles of going away to school and being away from home for the first time, living in a dorm with other girls who don't understand diabetes or choosing to eat healthy, and keeping up with the heavy course-load of a nursing student, in addition to working part time as a CNA while still in school, she continues to step up her game. Watching her grow from the passive, nonchalant girl she once was into the tenacious, progress-oriented young woman she is today brings me a sense of fulfillment that is hard to put into words. She inspires me every day to continue finding ways to grow, improve, and inspire others, and has truly become the little sister I never had. Check out her chapter contribution at the end of the book!

Testimonial: *"Before meeting Daniele, I would say I knew the basics of diabetes: test, eat, insulin. My A1cs were in the 9s and I just didn't really know how to manage my diabetes. Then Daniele showed me how to eat healthier and actually like it! She also gave me realistic goals about how to become healthier. I went from hardly taking care of myself, to being conscious of every decision I make and thinking of how it will affect my health. And not only was she there to teach me, she supported me and helped me along the way. Daniele has become one of my role models, who truly practices what she preaches. She has continuously shown me that you can accomplish what you set your mind to."* -- *Shay Leahy, 21, T1D, Hatboro, PA*

Shay's Mom, Kathy

When we step up and begin taking the steps to embrace our powers of choice, self-love, community, and action, amazing things begin to happen, not only within ourselves, but also in every other aspect of our lives. This includes our relationships with our family, friends, and significant others. Check out what Shay's mom, Kathy, has to say about the differences she has noticed over the years.

Testimonial: *It's hard to put into words, let alone a few sentences, the impact that Daniele has had on our lives. My daughter was diagnosed at the age of ten with type 1 diabetes. Until she hit puberty, her diabetes was manageable. When she turned 14, her diabetes spiraled out of control. A1c's that were previously in the low 7s were now in the high 9s. She gained weight and her attitude was miserable. Daniele entered her life when she was 16, and within a few months of working with Daniele every week, I felt like I had my daughter back. Daniele not only worked out with her, she counseled her on eating habits and making the right food choices. Daniele helped her plan out meals and created a realistic diet plan for a teenager. Having diabetes herself, Daniele could relate to the issues my daughter was having with being different from her friends. Daniele provided support and guidance. Daniele was always available for phone calls from me whenever I had questions or needed advice on how to handle an issue that arose from having a teenager with diabetes. Even though my daughter is now in college, she continues to meet with Daniele on a regular basis. Her A1c is back in the low 7s and she maintains a healthy weight, all thanks to her and Daniele's efforts!* --*Kathy L., mother of T1D client Shay, Hatboro, PA*

Rich

When I first began meeting with Rich, who has type 2 diabetes, he weighed 202 pounds and his A1c was in the 9s, close to 10%. Now, five years later at the age of 67, he weighs 170 pounds and keeps his A1c around 7%. According to Rich, his golf game has improved immensely, and now he gives the younger guys a run for their money. We still meet twice a week for maintenance workout sessions and diabetes management strategies, because in the realm of Diabetes Domination, accountability is key. He is an inspiration, one of the kindest people in the world, and a wonderful example of what you can do to change the quality of your life, no matter what your age.

Testimonial: *"Working with Daniele after having bypass surgery has really helped me to improve my strength and blood sugar levels. I have reduced my insulin by four units so far. The best part is that my golf game has improved dramatically! I'm giving the younger guys a run for their money now!" --Rich L., 67, T2D, Plymouth Meeting, PA*

Judy

One of my favorite success stories comes from very close to my heart, my Aunt Judy, who is now 80 years old. She took nightly injections of Lantus in addition to her oral medication. She lives in Las Vegas, so we don't talk as often as I would like (my fault), but whenever we do talk, we spend more than an hour on the phone, and one of our favorite topics of conversation is health. Early in 2012, we had a particularly intense conversation where I told her very specifically what she needed to do to feel better, have more energy, and to dominate her diabetes, because she was complaining about how she had been recently suffering through frequent swings in her blood sugar levels, going from low to high and back down quickly, and she couldn't understand why. This was also affecting her sleep schedule and overall quality of life. Long story short, she currently takes NO INSULIN at all. When she called to tell me that she was thrilled to take the Lantus out of her nightstand, the excitement and pride in her voice was indescribable, and I couldn't help but to cry tears of happiness for her. She told me that if she had continued listening to her doctor's advice, she would still be struggling with her nightly injections and constantly worrying about the highs and lows. It truly warms my heart to know that I was finally able to influence the habits of my favorite aunt. At 77 years old, she decided to change, to take control of her choices, and I was lucky enough to be a part of that.

Testimonial: *"After speaking with Daniele on the phone, I began following her instructions to the T. I just had enough of being out of control and feeling so tired all the time. I stopped taking insulin injections COMPLETELY."* --Judy P., 80, T2D, Las Vegas, NV

Donna and Sarah

Talk about a dynamic duo. These ladies took the proverbial bull by the horns and took diabetes head on. They work so well together and I immediately felt like I was a long lost part of their warm, welcoming family. They have come so far in such a short time, and Sarah's last A1c was 6.8! I couldn't be more proud of these incredible, strong women. Sarah is now a senior in high school and on her way to a limitlessly successful future.

Testimonial: *"While working with Daniele, I learned how to improve myself both mentally and physically. I learned how to build up my positive thoughts and boost my confidence all the while building up my muscles and living a healthier life. Her guidance really makes a difference and stays with you in the future. I am so happy to have been a part of such a successful program and I can't thank Daniele and my mother enough for their unwavering support."* – Sarah

"Some dates you never forget – birthdays, anniversaries, graduations, and then there's the day your child is diagnosed with type 1 diabetes. For us, that day was 06/08/13. Sarah was 14 1/2 at the time. Although I work in administration for a primary care physician's office and we see tons of diabetics, what I knew about diabetes was basically by default. I soon found out that what I THOUGHT I knew about diabetes was NOTHING compared to what I learned from Daniele. Life is hard enough on a good day. I am a hardcore optimist no matter what the situation is. So once we got the diagnosis, I was determined we would make the very best of the situation as soon as the shock wore off. Type 1 diabetes gives you about 5 minutes to figure out what the heck just happened and how to manage it. You feel like you've just been shot out of a cannon. There were many days when our worlds collided, emotions would explode because I thought Sarah was being irresponsible, and she thought I was being a hard case (to put it lightly). Although I know she was old enough to understand the complications, I wanted her to do things the way I wanted without stopping to

think how she was feeling. I felt like it was my mission to save her. Teenagers are funny (not funny) creatures and I had to back off a bit. I felt like I lived on the internet trying to find that "thing" that was just going to be the "aha" moment...and after 2 years....I found it. I needed to find someone that was diagnosed young, had experience weight gain, emotional stress, but through it all came out on top positive, healthy, and in great shape mentally and physically. Her name is Daniele Hargenrader. I was immediately impressed after reading her bio and knew I had to connect with her.

After we had our initial phone call I knew she was the one to help us get on track. Daniele's guidance, encouragement, incredible knowledge, and just overall awesomeness enveloped you like a big warm hug and you felt the fear, anxiety and worry start to melt away because you knew you had someone on the same journey with you that would not leave you. Parents need to feel that warm hug too sometimes. We try so hard to take the fear and anxiety from our children that it overwhelms us and can make matters worse. Daniele taught me as a parent that it's okay if Sarah misses the mark as long as she learns from it. She praises your good days, and encourages your not so great moments and turns them into learning experiences. Fighting diabetes is very mental for everyone involved. If you can keep it positive between the ears, the rest is a lot easier to manage. Understanding how food affects the blood sugars, how blood sugars affect everything else, having a positive mental attitude, knowing that achieving your goals will take time, loving yourself, and having someone guide you through it all that takes a personal interest in you is just a small portion of what makes working with Daniele the total package. We are not where we want to be yet, but we're a long ways from where we were. Taking it a day at the time and knowing Daniele will always be there is priceless...she will always be part of our family." - Donna

3

THE CHALLENGE

"When something is important enough, you do it, even if the odds are not in your favor."
-Elon Musk

I know that we've all heard this before, but some things are worth repeating: it has been said that insanity is doing the same thing over and over again and expecting to get different results. Sticking with our goals even after we go through failure/experience is admirable. What isn't admirable is trying to reach those same goals again without reassessing, and changing course a bit. There is strength to be found in mapping out a few different routes to reach our desired destination, just in case we hit a road block. After rerouting (aka picking ourselves up, dusting ourselves off, and keeping it moving forward), we will almost always find the success we seek, but almost never without going through the experience of failure first. Obstacles are to be expected in life, and as long as we set out on the path to success with that in mind, we will be prepared for them when they arise, instead of running into that wall and letting it be the end of our journey. As Josh Shipp says, "Perseverance is stubbornness with a purpose."

Reaching our goals will not be easy; if it were easy, everyone would be blissfully happy with their health and wellness. However, as life often teaches us, it is the obstacles and challenges that we overcome that build our strength and character, and show us what we are truly made of. When we think back over the course of our lives, there is most likely not a single one of us who got to where we are today unscathed by unforeseen obstacles. For me, without the obstacles of deep depression over the loss of my father, a binge eating addiction, the loss of my sister through drug addiction, and an outlook on life that told me I would be dead by 50, I would not be sitting here writing this book. I would not have the strength to help others embrace their personal power. I would not be me, and you would not be you, and we would not be us without the obstacles life inevitably puts on our paths.

If I didn't fail time after time, I would not be in the best health, shape, and mindset of my life, having type 1 diabetes for just under 25 years. I would not be able to share my experiences (failures) with you, the readers in our community, in hopes that you can and will learn from my mistakes so that you don't have to continue putting your body through the detriment that I did for so long. Please trust me when I say that all of our failures up until this point have been beautiful, valuable lessons. They have provided us with so much insight and hindsight and future foresight that is readily available to us at any given moment, and the sooner we allow ourselves to view it that way, the better off we will be. Our failures, obstacles, and challenges are part of our arsenal in the battle against our past bad decisions and judgments. Let's use them wisely, for they can either break us or build us up into an unstoppable Diabetes Dominator. The CHOICE is always ours to make.

4

MY STORY OF DIABETES DENIAL

"If you always put limits on everything you do, physical or anything else, it will spread into your work and into your life. There are no limits. There are only plateaus, and you must not stay there, you must go beyond them."
-Bruce Lee

Every good movie or book starts with a story of struggle, and this is mine. I was diagnosed with type 1 diabetes at the age of nine, in September of 1991, about three weeks after my birthday. Although, since I had been losing weight steadily and had all of a sudden began wetting the bed out of nowhere leading up to the diagnosis, it was apparent that I'd had diabetes for quite some time before actually being diagnosed. On top of those symptoms, I was always tired, insanely thirsty, urinating frequently, and had stomachaches almost every day. After being sent home sick from school two days in a row, my mom took me straight from school to the pediatrician's office. He recognized the symptoms and checked my blood sugar in the office, to find it was over 800.

I was immediately transferred over to the hospital, where we stayed for the next seven days. I say "we" because my mom slept next to me in that hospital room on a hard cot every single night, trying to grasp all of the new information that was coming our way, and comfort me as best she could. The internet was just a blossoming idea at the time, and my parents were scared out of their minds with the idea of taking the proper care of their child who now, all of a sudden, had an incurable disease that required around-the-clock monitoring and planning. We didn't have *Google* or cellphones (although my dad did have a car phone which I thought was the coolest thing ever, a tool essential to a travelling plumber back in the early 90s.) We didn't have these invaluable, endless networks of information at our fingertips. We didn't have the diabetes online community (DOC) in 1991.

The blood sugar testing was by far the worst thing for me at first. I had been taking violin lessons in elementary school for about a year prior to my diagnosis, but due to the incredible pain in all of my fingertips from the constant checking of my blood sugar, I had to give that up. I could no longer hold down the strings on the violin without being in pain. Back then, there was no exact readout from the glucometer in five seconds, either. First, you had to let your giant blood drop sit on a test strip for a minute, then wipe it off and put it in the machine. Another minute would go by, and then you had to take the strip out and look at what color it was and match it up to a color scale on the side of the test strip vial to best estimate in what range your blood sugar was. Thankfully, the methods we use to check our blood sugars have changed drastically in the past 25 years.

As a child, it's almost impossible to grasp such a deep and permanent change in your life, which is one of the reasons I think getting diagnosed at a younger age is easier for the child (but harder for the parents) to deal with, as opposed to getting diagnosed when you are older and much more set in your ways. All of a sudden, I was very different from all of the other kids. I had to eat at extremely specific times, inject myself with needles 3-6 times a day every day, and, most importantly, know what my blood sugar levels were at all times. Needless to say, this is more responsibility and knowledge than most nine-year-olds should ever have to bear.

As time went on, so did our lives. My mom was always a great cook and the one who prepared meals for our family, so she continued to do what she did best: be my mother, my caretaker, my champion, my rock. She invited me into the kitchen with her, showed me how to enjoy preparing food through her own enjoyment. However, this enjoyment didn't take hold right away; it wasn't until years later that my own love of cooking took over.

A few short years later, on August 25, 1994 (the day after my 12th birthday), our world truly came crumbling down. Our little family of three, who always had each other's backs through whatever adversity life put in our path, was suddenly and unexpectedly shattered. My father died of heart disease quite literally out of nowhere. Before this time, everything was "normal."

My parents had been blissfully married for 22 years before this awful, life-altering event took place. I say "blissfully" in total seriousness; they worked together during the day and came home together at night and never fought or got tired of each other. It was pretty amazing, now that I'm an adult and can think about it objectively. It was literally like we (my mom and I) had been blind-sided by a Mack truck going 100 mph. One month–hell, two weeks–before this happened, my father had been running the plumbing company that he co-owned and that my mother managed and did the bookkeeping for, going out on leads and coming back to the office where my mom kept everything in order.

The next month, he was dead, gone from our lives, just like that. He smoked cigarettes his whole life, starting at the young age of 12 and never stopping until his heart attack and death at the age of 55. He ate what he pleased, he was overweight, but there were no other external signs that we could identify leading up to this tragic event (not that smoking and eating an unhealthful diet weren't enough). After his heart attack, they performed an immediate quadruple bypass surgery at Hahnemann Hospital in Philadelphia, and he never recovered from the surgery. I never got to say "goodbye," or "I love you," or anything at all for that matter, due to the quickness that all of this took place. I remember sleeping in bed at home when the phone rang, and hearing the sound of my mom's voice on the other end, hearing her voice sound like I'd never heard it sound before. All she could say was "he's gone," and all I could say was "no" over and over and over again, somehow hoping that if I said it enough, what was happening would turn out to be just a horrible nightmare that I would eventually wake up from.

Needless to say, the sudden death of my dad, combined with diabetes and the onset of puberty, was more than enough leverage for me to give up on taking care of myself, specifically of my diabetes. I fell into a deep and dark depression, full of self-pity and rage, all fueled by the comfort I found in food, in eating whatever I wanted while I was alone in my home. In a short period of time, I blew up, both in weight and blood sugar/hemoglobin A1c numbers, until I was 200+ pounds and at an A1c of 13+%.

As I moved into my teenage years, diabetes became a more and more negative experience for me, as it is extremely difficult for a child/teen to be viewed as different from the other kids. It is hard for a child/teen to explain why they have to go to the nurse's office to eat a snack before lunch every day, and even when they try to explain, it is a very difficult concept for other children that age to understand.

It's hard enough to tell a kid that your pancreas isn't functioning properly when they don't know what a pancreas is. That pushed me further into my cycle of self-pity and detrimental rebellion.

I became more introverted and sad, and went through a phase where I didn't take insulin as I should have. I had a severe lack of self-control of my choices regarding my diet, lack of exercise, downward-spiraling self-image, and negative feelings of self-pity. As the number on the scale increased, so did my blood sugar readings, as well as my level of misery and depression–they were always directly proportional. I went from being an average-sized child to an obese teenager in short order. I was 12-13 years old, shopping in the adult women's plus-size section. Needless to say, I was beyond miserable and full of shame.

I felt completely out of control, helpless, hopeless, pitiful, and insane with anger: anger towards myself, towards the universe for dealing me this hand in life. "Why me? What did I do to deserve this?" I asked these questions over and over again. It wasn't enough to have type 1 diabetes, I had to have my father taken away from my mom and me, and have our lives uprooted as well? These negative, backwards-thinking, non-productive questions were spurring me further and further into my own personal hell, a hell where my blood sugar was rarely under 200, often over 400, and for anyone who knows what that feels like, I'm sorry to hear it because it is truly one of the worst feelings in the world. However, that extreme negativity that at the time, I thought would be part of my life forever, ignited a flame that has grown steadily over the years into a raging, fiery passion for the quest for any and all knowledge available regarding nutrition, physical fitness, psychology, diabetes, and the best ways to control our choices around those areas of our lives.

Food had become my comfort. My mom had to find a new full-time job to support us now that my father was gone; working at the plumbing company was just too painful for her, and understandably so. This arrangement mostly left me by myself after school. This was my opportunity to binge in private. I would take the bus home and get off early to stop at Wawa (think 7-11) or the local pharmacy. Here, I would buy whatever I wanted with my allowance, and go home and eat in the privacy of my own living room directly in front of the TV. It wasn't always Wawa, it was McDonald's and the like as well, really whatever I wanted that day, that minute. This also included things like cereal and milk, gummy snacks (Gushers, Fruit Roll-ups, etc.), Skittles, frozen bagels with cheese on them, granola bars, the list could go on and on. I pretended I didn't even have diabetes, that it wasn't even a thing I needed to pay attention to.

Although I had no idea back then, these events were shaping my teaching techniques for the future. For example, one of the first things I talk about when giving speeches to parents of newly diagnosed children or to people with diabetes struggling with weight issues is how NOT to create a dependency on junk food as the answer to low blood sugar. Instead, ONLY ALLOW 100% juice boxes, glucose gel, or glucose tabs for the treatments of low blood sugar, nothing else. Hypoglycemia is a medical emergency and should be treated as such. Using junk food as a reward or an excuse to have a "treat" in any scenario will have detrimental long-term effects in creating a hard-to-break habit of "rewarding" ourselves when our blood sugar is low.

I experienced my first hypoglycemic seizure in my sleep at the age of 14. I remember seeing my mom kneeling over me on the floor as I groggily awoke from the shot of glucagon she had given me. I was on the floor because as I was having the seizure, I fell out of bed and actually cracked a vertebrate in my lower back. Then came the ambulance and the visit to the hospital. That scared me in a way I'd never experienced before. That experience was the first time I really began thinking about what I was doing to myself, but it didn't make me stop my detrimental habits immediately.

The second hypoglycemic seizure I had was again in my sleep, while I was 16 years old and vacationing down the shore (Philly/Jersey language here!) with my older half-sisters and my cousin. I remember them pouring juice in my mouth and me coming to, completely confused and seeing them looking like they had just seen a ghost. I also remember feeling like the biggest burden on my family, and that surely nobody would ever want to go on vacation with me ever again. The third and final time this happened, and what was truly a turning point for me in the sense of reevaluating my health habits and figuring out who I was as a person and who I wanted to be as I was coming into adulthood, was when I was 17 and at a sleep-over at a friend's house, where there were four other friends as well. All I remember from that one was waking up in a hospital emergency room, confused and afraid, seeing my mom looking over me and wondering how I even got there; I didn't even remember the ambulance ride.

So many apologies to my friends' parents. So much shame. So much self-loathing and blame. So much feeling like an incredible burden on all the people I knew and loved. So much that I knew I couldn't continue living the way I had been for so long, ignoring my diabetes and pretending it would somehow just go away. Obviously, not only was it not going away, but it was coming out to haunt me more and more often, in more and more severe and life-threatening ways that were not only affecting me, but all those who surrounded and cared about me. It was time to change. For real this time.

5

MY JOURNEY TO LIBERATION THROUGH UNDERSTANDING, ACCEPTING, AND EMBRACING THE DIABETES DOMINATOR MENTALITY

"The only problem we really have is we think we're not supposed to have problems. Problems call us to higher level...Your past does not equal your future."
-Tony Robbins

Oftentimes in life, we need to go through bad times to truly appreciate the good; we need to experience pain to know the wonders of joy; we need to have consistently high blood sugars to know how good it feels to have blood sugars in a normal range. Going through my teenage years as an obese person with a binge eating addiction, ignoring my diabetes was a negative experience to say the least, but often when we have painful experiences in life, we are given the gifts of lessons learned, perspective, and experience. Now that I look back on those years, I know that I have those experiences to thank for making me who I am today, and who I am today is the Diabetes Dominator.

The Diabetes Dominator is not only a mentality, but a persona, a superhero identity who proudly wears his/her cape and knows that just living day-to-day with any chronic disease makes us superheroes. My quest for knowledge has led me to obtaining a Bachelor's degree in nutrition science, and led me through extensive training as a personal chef, diabetes coach, health coach, personal trainer, and meal planner for those with special medical needs. It has also spurred me to attend NPTI (National Personal Training Institute) to become a certified personal trainer. All of these experiences have been integral in shaping my ability to dominate my diabetes and help others do the same for themselves.

Through my many trials and tribulations while living with type 1 diabetes, I have come to many conclusions; however, the strongest and most important one is this: YOU and only YOU have the ability to dominate your choices regarding your diabetes care. We cannot control diabetes, but we can control the choices we make regarding our health and wellness habits which ultimately shape our reality. There is no severity level of diabetes. Either we have diabetes and choose to take good care of ourselves on a consistent basis, or we have diabetes and choose to take poor care of ourselves and neglect our health, making it a low priority in our lives (some people like to default to describing themselves as having "severe" or "bad" diabetes, when in reality, their symptoms of living with diabetes are more severe due to consistently poor choices with diet and exercise).

To some, this might sound harsh, but as cliché as it sounds, the truth does set us free. As soon as we become honest with ourselves and fully admit that we are in control of the food we put into our mouths and the way we move or don't move, the sooner we will feel empowered to step up and make the choices that we know will better serve our bodies, minds, energy levels, and overall health. To be clear, I'm not saying that taking these steps in the right direction will be easy, but I can promise that when you start seeing (and feeling) your blood sugar levels in the 100s instead of the 200s, 300s, 400s on a regular basis, the feeling of empowerment, freedom, accomplishment, confidence, and energy will make it much harder to go back to old patterns of self-destruction. Plus, if you struggle with weight-related issues, when you see those pounds start to drop off due to consistent healthy choices and actions, you will be in what I like to call an upward-spiral, and it is easy to get addicted to feeling happy, energetic, proud, strong, confident, and powerful. And speaking of energetic, our energy levels are one of the first things to change when we begin consistently choosing healthy foods and moving more often, not to mention getting much higher quality sleep, which is one of the most important aspects of our health.

Change usually comes from one of two things: inspiration or desperation. As Brendon Burchard says, "Either something new comes into our lives, or something new comes out of us." That is exactly what happened to me, more on the side of desperation. One day, being obese and constantly feeling tired, depressed, out of control of my health, and feeling like a burden on those who loved me became too much to bear, and it was like a light switch was flipped on in my head. I began reading and researching about all different kinds of diets, and tried them out. Some were more successful than others, but I was learning so much about how the human body works, about how my body reacted to different foods and different kinds of movement that I was actually enjoying myself.

I became a scientist, able to adjust my insulin depending on what I ate, which is at the top of the list of must-have skills to possess as a person living with diabetes. I also started taking an interest in exercising. Just to be clear, I'm not talking about the kind of exercise where you are dripping with sweat and can barely breathe (although I'm certainly not downing anaerobic training). I am talking about simple, easy things like walking (inside on a treadmill or outside), dancing around my living room to my favorite songs (or today, Zumba classes), elliptical machines, yoga, etc., all performed at a pace that while doing it, I could easily hold a conversation with a friend if I wanted to (aerobic training).

Slowly but surely, the weight started coming off, and that was over 10 years ago. Now, 24 years after my diagnosis, I feel happier and healthier than I ever have before, with the intention of always keeping it that way. I choose to be happy even when things don't go my way. Of course, there are days when I don't feel like dealing with diabetes. There are days when I want to pig out and eat anything and everything I want. But as we grow stronger, those days become rarer, and when they do happen or when my blood sugars aren't where I want them to be, I don't beat myself up.

I give myself credit for living with diabetes every day, and say that tomorrow will be a better day. We all deserve immense credit for living with diabetes, not only us, but those who care for and about us as well. Perfection is not a real, attainable thing, so it isn't something I ever aspire for. Instead, I aspire for progress. For more wins than losses. And for when I do experience what I perceive to be a loss, I don't berate myself for not being perfect, but rather examine the data I do have and see where I can make different choices the next time around. A happy, fulfilling life with diabetes (or without) is about progress, not perfection, and knowing that we are worthy and valuable individuals with a voice that deserves to be heard…every single one of us.

I have now reached a point in my life where my desire for knowledge has taken on a new direction and become not only a quest for knowledge, but an inherent need to share my experiences with others living with diabetes, as well as with our caretakers, our friends, families, and loved ones. After everything I have been through, all of the ups and downs, successes and failures, I have extracted the lessons learned from each experience in order to add value to others' lives so that they don't have to blindly guess their way through these situations, but can instead learn from my mistakes. It is one of my greatest joys in life to know that I have the ability to help so many people all over the world who struggle with diabetes, and I look forward to any and all feedback, questions, comments, stories, and experiences that will help me help you, and ultimately, help us help each other through our incredible diabetes community both on and offline.

6

YOU CAN DO IT TOO… WE ALL HAVE THE POWER WITHIN US

"Don't let someone else's opinion of you become your reality."
-Les Brown

Why should you adopt the Diabetes Dominator mentality? That is an answer that only you can provide. As my mentor Napoleon Hill said, "Many people learn the principles of healthy living, but do not develop the habits of applying them. We lose our inspiration, we stop trying. Motivation (an inspiration to action) is like a fire: unless it is constantly refueled, the flame is extinguished." The main reason I continue to refuel my flame of habitually applying the principles of healthy living is freedom.

Liberation from all of the endless BS that we hear every day in the media, and unfortunately even sometimes from our own doctors, family, friends, and online community about how horrible life is for people with diabetes. These are other peoples' opinions, nothing more. There is so much doom and gloom out there, so many unrequested opinions, and so much of it just isn't true unless we choose to allow it to be. I decided (as much as humanly possible) to liberate myself from the fears and insecurities of false or generalized information, as well as to liberate myself from the fears I had about taking my diabetes care into my own hands. We may have a chronic illness, but that doesn't mean we have to remain chronically ill prepared.

I have never felt more confident and empowered about every decision I make, every bolus I take, every carb I eat, every calorie I burn. It's all under my control, it's all by my own choice, and I know how to make the right decisions for myself by consciously and proactively using the data I have via the information and signs my body sends me. By using the numbers on my meter and CGM, by making my health and wellbeing my number-one priority so that I can give the best possible version of myself to everyone with whom I interact. We have to learn to prioritize our health so that we can give all and not just part of ourselves and all that we have to offer to the world. Wouldn't you like to feel confident and empowered about every diabetes-related decision you ever make for the rest of your life? You can do it, too.

3 Untruths that Damage Our Diabetes Community that We Have the Power to Change Together

1. All people with diabetes will have other health complications because of diabetes.
2. It is more important to concentrate on separating people with diabetes by type, to put ourselves into different categories, versus coming together as one strong group so that we can have a stronger voice in the patient advocacy world (more on this in a later chapter).
3. People with diabetes are limited in their ability to live their lives fully, realize their dreams, live out their passions, and participate in the day-to-day activities that those who don't have diabetes are able to perform.

Have you ever noticed that almost everything we ever hear about diabetes is negative and leaves us feeling worse than before we sought to learn something new? One of my biggest goals is to effect change in that system of messaging from the inside out. The power of suggestion is a very strong influence on the human brain, so when we hear about the many complications of diabetes, such as amputations, cardiovascular disease, kidney and liver failure, retinopathy, etc., it is unfortunate that the information provided is not more specific.

These are the complications that arise from consistently high blood sugars, from uncontrolled choices, not simply having diabetes. This omission of information leaves many of us convinced that we are doomed to suffer these complications solely based on the fact that we have diabetes, which simply isn't true! This drives me insane, as we live in a world where we need positive, forward thinking, constantly-learning, action-oriented, passionate leaders out to serve humanity who can inspire people to step up and be all that we can be instead of leading us into a life of complacency and acceptance of our inevitable fates.

Diabetes will only be the death of us if we so choose, and we always have a choice; every single action we take is a choice. EVERY SINGLE ACTION OR INACTION IS A CHOICE. Getting out of bed in the morning is a choice. Brushing our teeth is a choice. Running a 5k is a choice. Eating a pint of ice cream is a choice. Taking insulin is a choice (as long as we have access to medication). Checking our blood sugar is a choice (as long as we have access to supplies).

Even when we don't have immediate access to the things we need (which I have a lot of personal experience with), we can choose to take actions to increase our probability of getting what we need. Not doing any of those things are all choices. Once we become aware of our incredible powers of choice and action, once we awaken to that as our reality, we will never view our relationship with diabetes the same way again. More on the other two untruths coming up later in the book!

7

THE DIABETES DOMINATOR
SYSTEM EXPLAINED

"Each journey starts with the first step."
-Chinese Proverb

The system I've been able to create through all of my struggles and triumphs living with T1D for the past 24 years, as well as the incredible successes I've shared with my clients, has an easy-to-follow framework that I will lay out in this book step-by-step. This framework will allow anyone who is willing to put in the work to integrate these actions into their mind and body, and to synthesize them in whatever way works best in order to make them individualized, sustainable, life-long habits. The goal of the framework is to eliminate confusion about what actions need to be taken, so that when these steps are consistently put into practice, measurable progress in all areas will be the result.

The great thing is that each pillar feeds into the next, each having positive, noticeable effects on the others. I chose the word "pillar" to describe each area because it creates an image and a feeling of holding up a foundation. Each pillar in this system is meant to support the foundation of creating our own, sustainable healthy lifestyle habits that, once learned and integrated, are part of our awareness forever. And once we experience how it feels to be healthy and confident by understanding, accepting, and embracing these six pillars, it becomes much more difficult to slip back into our old, unhealthy patterns.

We do best when we set realistic expectations and set ourselves up for success. We are after small, permanent, attainable changes that will lead to huge differences down the road. I can't stress enough that this system will not work overnight. Whatever unhealthy habits we have fully integrated into our lives did not develop in a week, and we cannot realistically expect them to change that quickly. Truly, patience is a virtue here, and a gift that we all deserve to give ourselves.

It is so important to remember that we need to celebrate every single achievement, and there is nothing too small to be celebrated. That is how we set ourselves up for success, and continue to have the inspiration and motivation to move forward. Celebration is essential; allowing ourselves to feel successful as often as possible is crucial. Our brains are set up to enjoy and anticipate celebration. There is no better way to develop habits than to celebrate every little (or big) win we experience.

The Six Pillars of Health that Shape the Diabetes Dominator Mentality: Mindset, Nutrition, Exercise, Support, Body Systems, and Mindfulness.

Mindset: Our mindset is the beginning and ending of every single thing we ever do. Not preparing ourselves to have the right mindset before setting out on a mission is like going on a road trip in a foreign country where we can't read the street signs and expecting to just magically get to our destination. However, more often than not, that is how we set out to reach many of our goals, essentially self-sabotaging and setting ourselves up for failure. The bottom line is that with a plan (or lack thereof) like that, we will never get where we are trying to go, and, even worse, will end up frustrated, angry, and feeling more hopeless than when we began. This is why "mindset" is listed first. Nothing great ever gets accomplished with a bad attitude and a negative, unprepared mindset.

Nutrition: Once we get our minds right, the next thing we will need to focus on is what we consistently choose to eat and drink. The foods we eat and the liquids we drink are the fuels we use to help 11 completely separate but intertwined major systems inside of our endlessly amazing human bodies to work efficiently all at the same time to keep us alive and functioning optimally. This is something that I think we not only take for granted, but often don't ever give a second thought to.

When we consistently choose processed foods, sugary drinks, and diet sodas sweetened with harmful chemicals that the body is not made to process (I used to be insanely addicted to diet soda), it is like using duct tape to hold the bumper onto a car. It will hold for a while (and it might even be a long while), but eventually the tape won't be able to withstand the pressure and the bumper will fall off at any random moment, much like how our bodies will slow down—or worse, shut down—any of those 11 systems when it doesn't have the proper fuel to keep them going.

I love food. I love to cook and I love to eat. But at the end of the day, we must differentiate food from being a reward or a comfort to the fact that it is the fuel that keeps us going. What we consistently put on the inside of our bodies will be directly reflected on the outside, whether we like it or not.

In the nutrition section, I will not solely suggest that we give things up; instead, I will suggest awesome options that may not previously have been on our radar to replace the things that we need to ingest much less of to get healthy. It's not about depriving ourselves of things we like; it's about replacing them with healthier options that, nine out of ten times, the people I've worked with loved even more than what they were eating before.

Exercise: The human body was made to move. When we deny our bodies something as essential as regular physical activity, there is no way we won't feel the negative effects. Things like low energy, stiffness, aches, pains, sore joints, headaches, mood swings, depression, and so much more can often be lessened immensely, or even eradicated completely, with consistent movement 4-5 times a week. Exercise simply makes us feel better, no matter what our issues are.

When we move, we release endorphins that tell our brains we are feeling good, that's why some people describe having an "exercise high." Eventually after enough consistency, (most of the time) exercise will no longer feel like a chore, but rather a blessing to be grateful that we are able to do. To say that we don't have time to exercise is just an excuse, albeit the most popular one of all-time. Telling myself this (quite literally talking to myself out loud, like a mantra) when I don't feel like exercising is effective most of the time: there is someone out there right now who is much busier than you are, who is taking the time to move the one and only physical body they are gifted with in this life, because they know that if they don't, they will suffer the physical, mental, and emotional consequences, and because they know they will not regret it and feel so much better when it's done.

If we watch just one 20-minute TV show a day, that proves beyond a doubt that we in fact do have time to exercise, we are just choosing not to. Choosing not to exercise is like having an (insert car of your dreams here), leaving it sit in the garage 364 days out of the year, and expecting it to run like a dream when we eventually do turn that key and want to take it out for a spin. The same goes for our bodies; they won't run when we want them to unless we keep up with the routine maintenance.

Support: Although I didn't set out with the intention to follow a car analogy theme here, it seems to be working, so I will stick with it for now. Support is paramount in our success at liberating ourselves from the perceived shackles of living with diabetes. I find that, among the vast amount of people with diabetes with whom I get the chance to interact, one of the most common threads between us is that we don't know or get the chance to interact with other people who understand what it's like to live with diabetes on a regular basis (or at all).

To deny that we need a support team who we can turn to for assistance, advice, comfort, and love is like having our car break down on a road in the middle of nowhere and saying that instead of calling a tow truck (or roadside assistance), we are just going to push it indefinitely until we come to a service station. My point is that without support, we will eventually run ourselves ragged, and increase the physical, mental, and emotional damage trying to take on every aspect of diabetes management by ourselves.

Nobody can make the best decisions on changing our medications based on our specific, individual daily activities, except for ourselves with the advice of our doctors/CDEs/medical team, if needed. But others can help us put on our pumps or give us an injection now and then, and listen to our frustrations, even if the intent is not to fix them, but just allow us to express our feelings without judgement, maybe give us advice if we want it, and comfort and love us so that we know we are not alone. We all need this support.

Needing and asking for support IS NOT a weakness. Having the courage to ask for support is one of the biggest shows of strength we as human beings can display. Putting ourselves out there in the diabetes online community in chat rooms, forums, and *Facebook* groups, for example, and actually speaking up about what we need is a tough step for most of us. But choosing to take that first step can often be the beginning of incredible friendships that last a lifetime.

Chronic disease just isn't something one person is meant to manage alone. We need to swallow our pride and our fears and worries of being a burden or a bother to other people. We need to embrace the fact that we are all important, that we are all worthy of love and support, and that our voice deserves to be heard. We need to put in the effort to build our core support team so that when we do break down, so to speak, we know we can call someone to help us get back on the road as quickly as possible.

Body Systems: There are 11 major systems that are operating both independently of one another and in simultaneous harmony all of the time. These systems include our respiratory system, cardiovascular system, musculoskeletal system, digestive system, lymphatic system, and more. These systems that almost seem like magic, to which we don't have to give any particular commands, which allow our hearts to beat over 100,000 times a day even without our asking it to, all need some very basic, foundational support from us to operate and remain as close to homeostasis as possible.

These are things we often take for granted, like water, sleep, regular bowel movements (yes, we are going there!), and other things that affect these systems, like how we deal with stress and our varying energy levels, especially while living with diabetes. All of these things can and do affect our blood sugar levels, as well as our moods every single day. Understanding the basics about what our bodies need from us, and providing those needs to our bodies on a consistent basis can often greatly improve many health issues. In this book, we will learn the often overlooked and underrated foundational ways to love and care for our bodies, the one and only vessel we get in this life.

Mindfulness: Mindfulness is defined as "a mental state achieved by focusing one's **awareness** on the **present moment**, while calmly **acknowledging** and **accepting** one's feelings, thoughts, and bodily sensations." I love this definition because it clearly defines what it means to be mindful. All too often in our increasingly digital society, we continually become less and less mindful, not only of ourselves, our feelings, and the sensations that our bodies are sending us, but of the thoughts and feelings of the other people we interact with as well. How many times have we seen two or more people having a conversation while one or more of them is checking their phone, scrolling through social media sites, or just blatantly talking on the phone to someone else?

We've become so desensitized to this as a society that it seems normal to most people to half pay attention, to give half of ourselves to those we interact with. This mindlessness not only takes its toll on the relationships we have with others, but also on the respect we feel we deserve from others as well. One of the most important and often never addressed aspects of health and wellness is how mindful we are of our own actions, their consequences, our feelings, and how present we are in each moment, with both ourselves and those around us whom we love. The good news is that choosing to become more mindful each day, each moment, is just like any other habit. The more we practice, the more it becomes part of our habitual default behaviors.

The Diabetes Dominator System

By creating the Diabetes Dominator System, I've provided a clear-cut framework that, if followed consistently and integrated into our lives, has been proven time and time again to help us form and maintain sustainable habits. Join me and others in the movement to thrive with diabetes. Join us in dispelling all of these myths and untruths.

This system and its foundational pillars have allowed me to change my mind from "diabetes happened TO me" to "diabetes happened FOR me." For those of us who have had enough, for those of us who have reached our limit on negativity, doom, and gloom, and who desire to continue to prove that complications come from consistently high blood sugars (and not even always then, since I had consistently high blood sugars for many years and to this day do not have any diabetes-related complications), NOT just from diabetes alone, this is for us. For those who want to make these untruths common knowledge so we can reduce the fear of living with

62

diabetes and increase hope, inspiration, motivation, and aspiration. For those of us who want to help make these false beliefs a thing of the past, and spread the knowledge that teaches people that we can be in control of the choices we make about our bodies and our health.

We are not victims of diabetes! This system, if followed consistently, can and will reduce our A1cs, reduce the amount of insulin/medications we need to take, increase our overall energy levels, and for all people with diabetes who struggle with weight issues as I did for so long, following this system will help us sustainably shed body fat, too. We all have various opportunities throughout our lives to step up and make powerful choices. Just because we have a chronic illness does not mean that we must remain chronically ill prepared regarding the best ways to care for our health!

PART TWO - THE SYSTEM: UNDERSTAND, ACCEPT, AND EMBRACE THE DIABETES DOMINATOR MENTALITY

8

KNOW YOUR REASONS WHY

"The starting point of all achievement is desire."
-Napoleon Hill

Staying motivated. Seeking inspiration. Digging deep and finding determination. Taking action in the face of fear and doubt. Doing things we know we need to do to succeed in reaching our goals, even when we don't feel like it...ESPECIALLY when we don't feel like it. All of these things have one thing in common, and those are our reasons WHY.

There are no right or wrong reasons why, if they move us to great lengths. But we all must take the time to sit down, put pen to paper, and reflect on WHY we want to make changes to our health. WHY we want to change our relationship with our diabetes for the better. WHY we want to take control of our choices. WHY we deserve nothing less than the highest level of self-love and appreciation. WHY we will be willing to reach out to our community and seek help when we need it.

Over the years, I've been blessed to work with many clients, and one of the first things I ask is why they sought my help in the first place. The most immediate and surface-level answers are usually that they want to lose weight, have better A1c levels, learn how to eat healthier, want to incorporate exercise into their lives more consistently, or overall, they want to learn how to sustain a healthy lifestyle for the long run. Although these are all honest answers, these are not the true reasons why—they are all means to a much greater end.

After hearing any one of those responses, my next immediate question is, "Why do you want that?" That's when the silence usually sets in, because that is when the wheels really start turning. That's when the brain really starts searching for the answer to that seemingly simple, yet deeply profound question...WHY? Why do we want to lose weight? Why do we want to have better A1c levels? Why do we want to learn to eat healthier? Why do we want to exercise more consistently?

There are some answers that, when I hear them, let me know the person has, without a doubt, reached a breaking point and is ready to change. That the person has finally reached a point where staying the same is more painful to them than the thought of the effort required for change to take place. That the person needs to change almost as much as they need to breathe.

We, as human beings, are programmed to avoid pain. This is why, in order to truly change, we must have a high level of pain associated with staying in our current circumstances, which acts as a natural driving force that moves us to veer away from that pain by making changes. I know this because I went through this exercise and was asked the same question—"Why do you want to change?—before I began my journey to building a sustainable healthy lifestyle. My answer to that question, when I said it out loud, caused me to immediately break down into uncontrollable, hysterical crying, and I've never looked back since.

That reason why, that answer that causes chills to run through my body whenever I hear someone else say it is, "Because I want to live." All those other things—eating healthy, exercising, better A1c levels—they are all means to an end…because we want to LIVE. Because we know that if we don't begin to take control of those things, we are slowly contributing to our own demise, and that is an incredibly painful, uncomfortable realization.

When I had this realization, it was one of the most cathartic, overwhelming experiences of my life. I finally accepted that, for so many years, I had been choosing to actively contribute to my slow, emotionally painful death. And in those moments when my coach kept asking me why, why, why, why I wanted all of these things, I finally understood what he was after. He wanted to show me that all of those things I was listing, although noble goals, were not the reason WHY I wanted to be healthy. I wanted to live. I wanted to enjoy my life with my husband. I wanted to have an opportunity to have a family if I so chose. I didn't want my current choices to be the reason that those things might not be possible any longer.

Another hugely moving "WHY" that I've encountered over the years is that people also want to lead by example so they can influence their children to build healthy habits. They know their children will pick up their habits, whether they are healthy or unhealthy. Or, they want to be the best version of themselves so that they can physically and emotionally support their children or partner in ways they want to but are currently unable. One client told me that he wanted to be alive to walk his daughter (who was only six years old at the time) down the aisle one day; and he knew that if he continued to live the way he had been living up until that point, that would not be an option, and he could no longer bear to think about it for one more second. That is a "WHY" that is not a means to an end, but is in itself the end result for which we are looking.

Over the years, my reasons why have grown. Now that I know without a shadow of a doubt that I want to live as long and healthily as possible, and I can't bear the thought of having my day-to-day choices be the reasons why that might not be possible, and have put in the consistent work to make that who I am, I have changed as a person, down to my core, down to my soul. Now, the reasons why I choose to keep up the sustainable healthy lifestyle that I spent so many years building are kept alive for other reasons. Now that I have been on both sides of things—seen the darkness and lived in the hopelessness and defeat for so long, and have seen what is possible, both for me and for others—my "WHY" is now so much bigger than me.

I want to lead by example; I need to lead by example. I want to change the way people view living with diabetes. I want to be someone living with diabetes who is not a doctor, a CDE, or anything else other than a person, a peer, who lives a wildly passionate, healthy, successful life, full of self-love and appreciation, who chases her dreams with complete abandon. Someone whose love and desire to be of service to others is immeasurable. Someone who needs to stand up for her peers and help them find the voice they may have temporarily lost. I need to let my light shine as brightly as possible. I need to guide others to listen more closely to that voice inside all of us that I drowned out for so long that whispers, *there is more to life than this.*

And the reason WHY I need to do this is in the hopes that other people will see my light shining and, possibly after years of suffering and dimming their own light like I did, finally understand, accept, and embrace that they can also change their circumstances and shine their own light brightly on the world. As one of my mentors, Marianne Williamson, says, "As we let our own light shine, we unconsciously give other people permission to do the same." The only difference is that I am not doing this unconsciously. Something bigger than me has entered my life, some unseen force that I feel stronger and stronger in my heart every day.

I strive to fully and completely embrace this light of service that the universe has given me. More than once, I have had the indescribable blessing of feeling those feelings involved with witnessing someone else's light come on for the first time, through the vehicle of allowing my own light to shine, and I can never go back. This is my new reason WHY, and it is more powerful than I can ever explain. We all have this light inside of us. Every single one of us has the power to "go confidently in the direction of our dreams, and to live the life we imagined," as Henry David Thoreau so eloquently put it more than 150 years ago.

So, what is your WHY? What are your reasons WHY? This is an exercise that could take some time to get to the bottom of; or, conversely, could open up a floodgate of reality against which you might have built up a huge dam for so long that, as soon as you tap on it, will break down, and the real reasons WHY will come pouring out. Either way, this must be addressed. We must be willing to dig deep and be fully honest with ourselves.

That way, when we experience the failures and setbacks that are inevitable on any journey to bettering ourselves and our circumstances, we will have our reasons WHY we started strong and determined to succeed to fall back on and to give us the push of reality that we will need to pick ourselves up, dust ourselves off, and keep things moving forward. Knowing our reasons why helps us embrace that every setback is a setup for a comeback. Knowing our reasons why helps us embrace that every failure plants a seed of equivalent opportunity; we just have to be willing to look for it. This is a crucial step that cannot be skipped, and I recommend doing it right now!

ACTION ITEM:

In your journal, write down your top three reasons WHY you want to change your relationship with diabetes. It can be helpful to think about what pain you've experienced in the past by not changing your relationship with diabetes, what suffering you are experiencing now, and what the consequences will be in the future—one, two, even five years down the road—if you don't begin to make changes now.

9

A GUIDING FRAMEWORK TO HELP US GAIN PERSPECTIVE: WHERE ARE YOU NOW, WHERE HAVE YOU BEEN, AND WHERE ARE YOU COMMITTED TO GOING?

"Every time you are tempted to react in the same old way, ask if you want to be a prisoner of the past or a pioneer of the future."
-Deepak Chopra

There are five categories that, over years of self-reflection and working closely with clients, I've identified regarding where we currently might be in our relationship with diabetes, and where it is possible to go. These categories make up the Guiding Diabetes Dominator Framework. After reading the outlines below, it is up to us to choose (with brutal honesty) where we are currently, followed by where we are aiming to go.

Category 1: Diabetes Denier: This category is unfortunately a place in which too many of us have chosen to live for too long (including myself). This could also be identified as "diabetes burnout." The characteristics of the Diabetes Denier include consistently choosing to ignore that our diabetes exists by actively avoiding checking our blood sugars, regularly choosing to eat and drink items that we KNOW are harmful to our bodies, avoiding exercise like the plague, and an overall feeling of hopelessness and defeat regarding our health and ability to manage our diabetes. Basically, we know we have diabetes, but choose to deny it and make no attempts at making small changes or progress in any way. This is

NOT a place that is fun to live in, believe me, I know. I lived there for almost ten years.

Category 2: Diabetes Darer: The characteristics of the Diabetes Darer include choosing to recognize that we have diabetes, and then committing to taking baby steps outside of our comfort zones on a regular basis. We find that this leads to our day-to-day lives being and FEELING more manageable, predictable, habitual, and routine. A Diabetes Darer has, at a minimum, a basic understanding of what must be done, and begins taking small, permanent steps (progress) towards forming long-lasting habits for optimal health whether they fully believe things will work out or not. A Diabetes Darer won't always follow through with the things they have decided to do, but they are consistently thinking about and maybe even venturing into planning out what needs to be done. Living in this framework slowly allows us to go a little further than before by incorporating those actions into our lives, feeling good about them, and being fueled to keep going by those feelings of accomplishment.

Category 3: Diabetes Decider: The characteristics of the Diabetes Decider include not only choosing to recognize and acknowledge our diabetes, but also consistently deciding to DO the things that need to be done, even when we are fearful and not sure we will succeed. Even when we don't feel like doing something, we do it anyway. As a Diabetes Decider, we are checking our blood sugars regularly, keeping a log of our food and water intake (much more to come on that later), and exercising three or more times a week. A Diabetes Decider has taken that daring attitude to the next level, even though uncertainty might be (and most likely is) present, they have decided to take action anyway. The habit might not be fully formed yet, but it's on the verge. It is at this point that we might begin to realize that diabetes allows us to understand at a profound level how precious our health really is, and how much control we really do have over it via our choices.

Category 4: Diabetes Doer: The characteristics of a Diabetes Doer include actually DOING all of the things mentioned in Category 3 CONSISTENTLY and CONFIDENTLY, feeling good about it, feeling proud of our discipline and results. A Diabetes Doer will also feel the pull to lead by example and to inspire others to aspire to be and do more for themselves, because we understand that we all deserve self-love, health, and happiness. Our health and energy levels will be at a record high, and the enthusiasm we have about our confidence in our abilities to intelligently track our daily diabetes management practices will be contagious. Others around us will notice our enthusiasm, confidence, and positive energy. Diabetes Doers might also feel the desire to add variety and intensity to their workout routines, as feeling stronger and more capable often does. Steadily getting stronger, feeling more empowered and confident, and being open and willing to embrace change means we are on the edge of the Diabetes Dominator mentality.

Category 5: Diabetes Dominator: The characteristics of the Diabetes Dominator include tangible, visible results, and also results that are hard to describe because we can just FEEL them as part of our being. When our A1c readings are consistently 7% or less, our energy levels are where we want them to be, and our relationship with our diabetes has truly been redefined, and something inside of us shifts. In order to achieve this, we have to be doing all of the things mentioned in Category 4; however, at this stage, it is part of who we are, part of our identity. These actions are much less of a struggle and more of an automatic reaction. We have not only fully understood and accepted that we have diabetes, but we have also embraced it.

Instead of fighting it, we have decided to dance with it, nurture it, and understand that we are ultimately in control of our decisions, and it is our decisions that shape our realities. We have also accepted and embraced the work that comes along with having diabetes, because we are truly passionate about creating and sustaining the best versions of ourselves, not just on occasion, but for life. The Diabetes Dominator mentality is accompanied by a strong desire to serve others and share our knowledge, passion, and love, in order to help empower other people to step into their own personal power and take control of their health-related decisions. All the things mentioned in previous frameworks have become deeply ingrained habits that are automatic; again, part of who we are. A Diabetes Dominator knows that diabetes isn't something that fuels self-pity and self-doubt but instead fuels self-love, self-care, self-appreciation, service, strength, empathy, and growth at levels we previously thought impossible and unattainable.

ACTION ITEM:

In your journal, write down where you think you are. Then decide where you want to be, even if you're not sure how you will get there just yet. Remember, this is just a guiding framework. Feel free to come up with your own categories!

10

THE INCREDIBLE IMPORTANCE OF GOAL SETTING, STAYING FOCUSED, AND TAKING ACTION

"The beginning of a habit is like an invisible thread, but every time we repeat the act we strengthen the strand, add to it another filament, until it becomes a great cable and binds us irrevocably, thought and act."
-Orison Swett Marden

No matter what framework we are currently operating in, in order to level up there are three specific things that need to be done ALL OF THE TIME, consistently. We must schedule these action items into our weekly plans (Sundays work best for me). This is the time when we write out our goals for the upcoming week, and revisit our goals from the past week.

This is the time when we choose what our primary focus and actions will be for the upcoming week. When we fail to plan, we plan to fail. Cliché I know, but always true nonetheless. Here is a bit more information on why choosing to incorporate this planning time into our lives is of ultimate importance, and how to get it done.

1. **GOALS**: We MUST set SPECIFIC GOALS, both for the short term and the long term (for example, weekly goals, 30-day goals, three month goals, six month goals, one year goals). These goals need to be kept in a spreadsheet of some sort, whether we use Excel, Google Drive (my personal favorite, because it is accessible from anywhere/any device), a piece of good, old-fashioned paper in a notebook or on a whiteboard that we can easily see and access every day. These goals need to be SPECIFIC. I know I keep saying that, and I promise you there is good reason for my repetition.

If you come up to me and say "I want to lose weight" and then we have a coaching session and one week later you've lost two pounds, technically, you have reached your goal, you've lost weight. Because the goal was so vague and you did in fact lose weight, your brain will stop supplying you with the motivation, inspiration, and focus to stay dedicated and continue taking action. Has that ever happened to you in the past? I went through it so many times, and often gained back the weight I lost, plus a few more pounds.

If you say "I want to permanently lose ten pounds in the next 60 days," that statement creates a crystal clear vision of what you are working towards, and an exact timeframe in which you are aiming to achieve it. This level of laser focus causes our brains to understand that the end result hasn't been achieved until it actually has, and we are much more likely to sustain our motivation, inspiration, and focus to take the actions required to achieve that goal. It is also super important to have new future goals already set before we reach any more immediate goal, so that our brains don't jump off the progress bandwagon.

2. **FOCUS** on these goals consistently. Make a vision board that you see every single day. Let these goals fill your thoughts with clear visions of what life will look like when you get to that end result. When we close our eyes at night, it is incredibly helpful to visualize ourselves AFTER we have reached our goals. We must see in our minds what we will look like, feel the feelings that we will feel when we achieve what we have set out to do, smell what life will smell like, taste the proverbial victory, engage all of our senses to KNOW what success looks and feels like to each of us, so that when we get there, we know that it's time to celebrate.

    We must breathe deeply as we focus on these thoughts, and connect them, or sync them up with our brainwaves and desires. Taking action to harness our focus is incredibly powerful. Make vision boards (these are incredibly powerful tools!), timelines, spreadsheets, trackers (again, I love Google

Drive for this so we can visually see our progress anytime, anywhere, and see how far we have come). I've said it before and I'll say it again: *"where your focus goes, your energy flows."* – Tony Robbins

Setting goals and harnessing our focus leads us to the third and most important thing of all…like seriously the most important thing ever…

3. **ACTION builds traction!** I'm sure you've heard people say that knowledge is power, but that isn't entirely true. Knowledge without ACTION holds very little power. How many things do we all KNOW that we should be doing for any number of beneficial reasons, but that we simply aren't taking the ACTIONS that we KNOW we need to in order to succeed? If we simply KNOW something but don't put that knowledge into practice by taking specific and directed ACTIONS, that knowledge is basically useless.

    "Common knowledge is not always common practice" -- Brendon Burchard.

    The easiest possible example is this: we all know that eating a whole foods plant-based diet full of foods that grow from the earth and are not processed out of their natural state, along with regular exercise and proper hydration, allows us to feel incredible and have excellent health. Quite literally, almost everyone in the world knows that, to some degree. But the vast majority of people are not actually doing it.

    The bottom line is: knowing isn't enough, we need to DO. We are all full of knowledge that we don't choose to put into action. That is the difference between successful people and unsuccessful people; successful people DO whatever needs to be done, regardless of whether they feel like doing it or not, because they KNOW that ACTION is the key to succeeding.

    An average person of average intellect who hustles and consistently takes action will beat out the lazy genius every single time. This could come in the form of one small action per week that we incorporate into our lives until it becomes a habit, and then picking another, slowly building a sustainable healthy lifestyle. For example, taking action to ensure that we are drinking half of our body weight in ounces of water every single day, and making sure it gets done by using a refillable water bottle and keeping track of the ounces.

Then the following week, take the necessary actions to incorporate five or more servings of vegetables into our diet every single day, and also take a couple hours out of the weekend to do a little basic planning and prepping. The goal is not to accomplish everything all at once and overload our plate with so many new actions that we are setting ourselves up for failure. Self-sabotage is the Diabetes Dominator's enemy, so be aware of this very human quality that we all possess and use far too often. Small, permanent steps turn into giant, sustainable results.

One other very important thing to keep in mind is that creating a sustainable healthy lifestyle and having a healthy relationship with our diabetes is a journey. The three steps we have to get through on any journey of change are first understanding, then accepting, and finally embracing. First, we must understand that our circumstances are not what we would like them to be, and that there are actions that we can take to change them. This is followed by accepting those actions as part of our daily routine, and really learning to make them habitual. The last step is embracing these changes as our new way of life. Sometimes these three steps happen really quickly. Other times, these steps take years to climb.

It took me many years to finally embrace my diabetes as a part of my life, a part of who I am that needs to be nurtured and cared for instead of being hated and dreaded. All those years of struggle and anger and fear that I went through before I was able to reach a place where I am now, at peace with my diabetes, were the original catalyst for the creation of the six pillars of total health system that I am going to cover in detail in the next sections. This system of how to essentially work through each of the most important aspects of our health is what I wish would have been available to me when I was depressed, angry, confused, and using food as my comfort, without a clear picture of where to start or how to make changes last. My genuine hope is that this system serves each reader the way it has served my clients and me for the past ten years.

ACTION ITEM: Take a few minutes right now to write out some of your goals. Maybe just for the next 30 days. Maybe you want to visualize what the next three months, six months, or one year could hold for you if you simply wrote down the things you want to achieve. There is incredible power in putting pen to paper and getting the things that are rattling around in our heads out into the universe.

Just seeing our goals, revisiting them each day, even if we don't know exactly HOW we will make them come to be, will make the likelihood of us reaching those goals increase a hundred fold. Letting our goals out of our heads makes them real. What do you want to be real in your life? When you unleash your goals from the confines of your brain out onto paper, the universe begins to conspire to guide you towards the "how" of getting it done.

11

THE WHEEL OF TOTAL HEALTH

"Progress is impossible without change, and those who cannot change their minds cannot change anything."
-George Bernard Shaw

Review the 6 Pillars on the Wheel of Health (on the next page). When filled out, the wheel is meant to create a current view of balanced health for you, and clearly demonstrate which Pillars need the most focus and attention giving you a blueprint of exactly where to get started to create your own sustained healthy lifestyle.

ACTION ITEM: Rank your current level of satisfaction HONESTLY with each pillar of total health by drawing a line across each segment using the scale from 1 to 5 that indicates where you think you are right now (1 = very dissatisfied and 5 = fully satisfied). This is meant to show a clear picture of how happy you currently are with each pillar of health in your life. You can either fill it on your page (don't be afraid to write on the book if this is a physical copy), or you can draw your own wheel in your journal. You can also get a copy of this wheel to print as many times as you would like at: **http://diabetesdomionator.com/thewheel**

1. Is your wheel moving you forward, keeping you from moving at all, or rolling you backward?

- MINDSET (BELIEFS, LANGUAGE, THOUGHTS, EMOTIONS)
- NUTRITION
- FITNESS
- BODY SYSTEMS (SLEEP, ELIMINATION)
- SUPPORT (ACCOUNTABILITY, MOTIVATION, CELEBRATION)

- MINDFULNESS (PAYING ATTENTION WITH INTENTION)

2. What does it look and feel like for YOU to be successful in each of these areas? Really take some time to think about your answers, and be very specific so that you know exactly what you are working towards and will immediately recognize it when you get there so you can CELEBRATE your success and sustain your motivation.

3. The perimeter of the circle represents your current 'Wheel of Total Health'…Is it a bumpy ride?

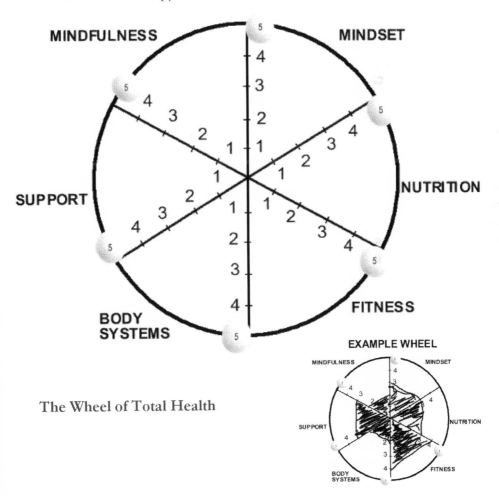

The Wheel of Total Health

Now, looking at the wheel, let's take this a little deeper and really get CLEAR on YOUR blueprint:

1. Are there any surprises for you?
2. How do you feel about your health and your life as you look at your wheel?
3. How do you currently spend time in these areas?
4. How would you like to spend time in these areas?
5. Which of these elements would you most like to improve first?
6. How specifically could you make space for these changes?
7. Can you effect the necessary changes on your own?
8. What help and cooperation from others might you need?
9. What would make each of the 6 pillars a score of 5 for YOU?
10. What would a score of 5 look like for you AS SPECIFICALLY AS POSSIBLE?

PART THREE - THE SIX PILLARS OF TOTAL HEALTH AND THE DIABETES DOMINATOR SYSTEM

1. Mindset
2. Nutrition
3. Exercise
4. Support
5. Body Systems
6. Mindfulness

12

MINDSET

"As you think, so shall you become."
-Bruce Lee

The reason I am addressing mindset first in the Diabetes Dominator system is because, at the end of the day, it's all in our heads. One of my favorite and most poignant quotes from t Tony Robbins that helped to change my mentality (and that I've mentioned already) is: "where your focus goes, your energy flows." Until I really integrated and synthesized exactly what that meant, it didn't mean anything to me; they were just words. However, I eventually realized that those words are the absolute reality-shaping truth for any and all aspects of life.

If we focus hard enough and consistently enough on something, think about it all the time, no matter if it's something we really DO want, or if it's something we really DON'T want, we will end up finding more of it manifesting in our lives. This is why it is of the utmost importance to recognize our very real power of choice and decision in all situations where we truly want to make sustainable changes and new habits to reach a goal or to create a lifestyle, specifically in directing our thoughts.

As human beings, what we focus on and the mindset in which we live most often are based on five main factors, all of which have different subcategories that are all within our control, whether we are aware of it or not.

- Our beliefs, meaning the things we are CERTAIN are true in life, and the meanings we assign to the things we experience
- Our emotions and feelings, meaning what we feel and why we feel that way, and our conscious use of our powers of gratitude and choice (choosing to be grateful, choosing love, choosing to ask for help, and choosing to let others in)

- Our physiology, meaning the way we move (or don't move) our bodies
- Our language, which directly shapes our thoughts and questions, meaning the words we use when we talk to ourselves and to others, and the words we use to describe things and situations which shape the questions we consistently ask ourselves, others, and the universe
- Self-sabotage, feeling overwhelmed, and failure, and how we deal with these inevitable aspects of life

Beliefs: A belief is something about which we have total certainty. The power of our current beliefs is strong, and is most likely the main reason we are not experiencing the quality of health and life that we desire at the moment. Our beliefs have been being shaped since early childhood by our external influences, including our parents, teachers, friends, family, media, as well as our personal experiences. And sometimes, as we get older and wiser, we might find that something we used to believe with total conviction now seems silly.

"It's not the events of our lives that shape us, but our beliefs as to what those events mean."
-Tony Robbins

Can you think of an example of something like that in your life? Something that maybe fifteen, ten, five, or even one year ago, you knew with absolute certainty was true, but now when you think about it, you know that not only was that belief false, but it wasn't serving you in any positive way? In fact, it was holding you back from being your true self, from living your best life. Everyone goes through these transitions in life. We have to be ready, willing, and able to admit that we were wrong, and be completely okay with that. Changing what we believe is normal, natural, human, and necessary. Change is the price of survival.

Here's an example from my life. When I was first diagnosed in 1991, the information I was given was pretty frightening. I was told in detail about the complications that were sure to arise over time, and that people who live with diabetes have, on average, a 15-year shorter lifespan than those who don't have diabetes. Since my father passed away at the age of 55, I assumed that put me at a lifespan of around 40, 50 if I was lucky.

So that was my reality, that is what I believed to be true with complete certainty for almost ten years before I railed against what I was told to believe, and formed my own new beliefs. From the time I was nine, until the time I was 19, I fully believed that I was destined to lose a toe (or two), destined to go blind, and destined to die by 40 or 50 years old. Those beliefs were just some of the many contributing factors that fueled my depression and my binge-eating problem that led to my obesity. I figured that if that was the way it was going to be, who cares what I eat or if I exercise, if I'm just going to suffer and die anyway?

Over time, I learned new information and found that I cared, my mom cared, my friends and family cared. I met new people who were kicking ass while living with diabetes. I saw more proof that what I had previously believed was simply not true. I was finally ready to admit that I had been so wrong for way too long, and that it was time to change. I had enough new information to decide that my old beliefs were complete BS, and, not only that, they were slowly killing me as well.

It was up to me, it was my choice to let these old beliefs go and re-define what I believed about living my life with diabetes. And so I did. I took what we all know as the "five Ws" and applied them to my current beliefs, and I suggest that you take the time to do so as well to get a much broader understanding of your beliefs and how to begin changing them to better serve your journey to health, self-love and self-respect.

ACTION ITEM – Five Ws: Remember that belief I asked you to think of a couple of paragraphs back? The one that, some time ago, you believed with total certainty, but that when you think about now seems almost absurd? Write that belief down on a piece of paper, then list the five Ws below it in order to clearly understand how that belief became one of your own.

- Who?
- What?
- When?
- Where?

- Why?

Who were the people who influenced me to believe that? What were the circumstances in my life going on at or around the time that I accepted that as a belief? When did I begin believing that? Where did that belief come from, and/or where was I in my life when that belief took hold? Why did I believe that for as long as I did before I changed my mind about what the truth really was? And why was I able to let it go and change my mind about what I believed?

Really do this exercise, I can't urge you strongly enough. When we take the time to dig deep into the recesses of our minds, going as far back as we can to truly discover the roots of some of our beliefs, the things we find out can often be surprising and incredibly liberating. Give yourself the freedom from some of the old, stale beliefs that may be holding you back from making the progress you desire and deserve!

Right this minute, I have no doubt that there are a number of beliefs that you have about yourself, your circumstances, meanings you've assigned to your experiences, other people, or the world in general that are holding you back from making progress, both with your quality of health and quality of life. Remember that there was a time when everyone believed without a shadow of a doubt that the earth was flat? That there was a time when everyone believed with 100% certainty that the sun revolved around the earth? These are just a couple of broad, worldview examples of the fact that having the ability to not only let go of old beliefs, but to replace them with new, empowering beliefs that are actually the truth constitutes real strength and character in an individual.

People who discover and share these new truths, as well as those who adopt them, are heroes, because they are going against the crowd, regardless of the consequences. The ability to step back and examine something that we once believed with total certainty and to admit that not only was it a belief that was holding us back, but that we are willing to let it go and make a new truth for ourselves is the ultimate use of our power of choice. I used to believe that diabetes was a curse that I had earned in a past life for doing something horrible, and that I would always be a closet binge-eater, because that was the state of my life for so long.

Now, when I look back at those horribly damaging beliefs and meanings that I created for myself, I know with 100% certainty that they were holding me back in a huge way and ultimately those were the things sending me to an early grave, not simply having diabetes. The TRUTH is that diabetes didn't happen TO me, it happened FOR me. If it weren't for diabetes, I would no doubt be as uninterested in and uneducated about the incredible importance of mindset, nutrition, and fitness as the general population of the world currently is, and most likely would have gone the way of many of my family members and stayed obese and unhealthy. The TRUTH is that I have an undeniable desire to eat clean, healthy, whole foods that grow from the earth and have not been processed into something else, instead of packages of cookies, endless bowls of cereal and milk, and fast-food, because I DESERVE IT! My body deserves to be treated with ultimate respect, as it is my only vehicle in this life, my temple. You, and your temple, deserve this too, whether you currently believe it or not.

ACTION ITEM: My challenge to you is to write down your current beliefs and meanings that you've assigned to events or experiences you've had that are holding you back or simply not serving you in a positive way regarding who you are (the way you think/act), your health (the way you take care of yourself/don't take care of yourself), and your reality, based on what you believe to be true with complete certainty. Then, challenge yourself to keep any beliefs that are definitely serving you and moving you forward, and cross out the ones that are holding you back. After you cross out the old ones that are keeping you from having the quality of health and life you desire and deserve, you MUST replace them with new truths – every single one of them. You should do this as often as you need to (once a day, once a week) until all of those self-deprecating, negative beliefs are eradicated, and you can recite your new truths from memory, because you know them to be true without any doubt. That is when you know you have fully integrated those new truths into your reality. I've included an example of this exercise below.

What I Believed Before:

I used to believe that I am too busy to plan and prepare my meals for the upcoming week ahead of time.

The Truth Now:

~~I believe that I am too busy to plan and prepare my meals for the upcoming week ahead of time.~~

The TRUTH is that TV, Facebook/Twitter/Instagram/YouTube, and other distractions that don't contribute to my health and wellness can wait. I am strong, committed, and determined to ensure that my body receives the nutrition it needs by taking 1-2 hours during the weekend to shop for and prepare foods for the upcoming week.

Emotions and Feelings: Our emotions and feelings have a direct effect on our beliefs and how we experience life in general. When we consistently feel certain emotions (what I refer to as "go-to" or "comfort zone" emotions), those feelings easily determine what we believe to be true, based on how things make us feel. Our emotions and feelings are all influenced by a few factors, all of which I've already talked about or will discuss soon: our physiology (how we intentionally use/position our bodies), our language, and our focus.

One of the biggest influences in my life, personal development coach, motivational speaker, and author Tony Robbins, has irrefutably taught me that emotion is created by motion. In fact, I hope you will try out this exercise to prove to yourself that this is true. When I first did this exercise, I was in a gigantic room in New Jersey, surrounded by a thousand other people, all of whom were, like me, trying to better understand our emotions. Trying to understand why we felt what we felt and acted the way we acted. Trying to figure out how we could choose certain ways of moving our bodies, use our physicality, to change our emotional state at the drop of a hat in order to help enrich our lives and get "unstuck."

It was at this seminar, this four-day live event in 2008 where I learned the tools that helped me understand and shape my emotional state (specifically related to my relationship with diabetes), and where the direction of my health and my life truly began to become a thing that I felt like I had a real handle on, for the first time ever. If I could change my emotional state any time I wanted to, I could do anything.

ONE MINUTE ACTION ITEM: For the next 30 seconds, take your eyes off this book and clear your mind as much as possible. Sit down, slump your shoulders forward, and bow your head. Sit this way for 30 seconds and just notice how you feel. Then, write down the first three emotions you felt during those 30 seconds.

Then, for the next 30 seconds, stand up with your shoulders back, chest up, and take deep, slow breaths while looking forward or even upward. Then, write down the first three emotions you felt during those 30 seconds. Compare them to the three emotions you felt in the other position. Don't put too much thought into this, just do it, pay close attention to how you feel, and see what happens.

If you're like most people in the world (this experiment has been conducted with over 30 million people, from almost all countries, at Tony Robbins' seminars), you probably noticed that when you were sitting down with your shoulders slumped forward and your head down, you felt some negative emotions, maybe even sadness or depression. But when you stood up, rolled your shoulders back, let your heart (chest) lead outward, and breathed deeply, you may have felt strong, capable, and resourceful. This is not a coincidence.

This shows us that the way we choose to position and use our bodies at any given moment directly influences the way we feel. There have been a plethora of scientific studies that have proven beyond a doubt that smiling and moving around (jumping jacks, for example), even when forced, produce lasting feelings of happiness (Google it, I promise this is true). However, just like anything else in life, this ability to change our emotional states won't work unless we practice, unless we consciously take action and choose to change how we are feeling at any given moment.

If I notice that I'm feeling negative emotions, or am feeling unproductive and just not accomplishing what I set out to do (anything from checking my blood sugar to making myself a quick meal to writing a book, and everything in between; nothing is too small or seemingly insignificant to use this valuable physiological tool on). The first thing I do is stand up, roll my shoulders back, and breathe deeply. Next, I focus on a thought that makes me happy (pets are a great tool here; petting my cats is an almost guaranteed instant warm and fuzzy feeling), followed by 30-50 jumping jacks, while smiling and thinking about that thought. The whole process takes under one minute; however, the end result will, nine times out of ten, involve feeling better than I did one minute before, and feeling inspired to do whatever it is I had been putting off.

I have one more tool that is the most powerful one of all when it comes to changing our emotional state, and I'm going to lay it on you in a minute. But first I'd like to share a few things about myself so you know that just like all of us out here in this crazy world, life isn't always rainbows and unicorns. In fact, sometimes it's pure hell. I know we all go through our own trials and tribulations in life, we are all dealt any number of crappy cards, but like Charles Swindoll's famous quote says: "life is 10% what happens to us and 90% how we react to it."

I'm not a cyborg (despite my various mechanical parts à la CGM and pump), I get angry, sad, and frustrated. I feel searing rage and I get depressed from time to time (although I haven't experienced the level of severe depression I experienced throughout my teenage years in about seven years). I recognize that feeling these emotions is okay and completely normal and acceptable on all levels. However, living with these emotions for any prolonged period of time is not acceptable for me, and once I realized that I had the power to change my emotions, I almost never let negative emotions rule my life for too long.

Depending on the catalyst for the negative emotions, I put a real and specific cap on when they will end, no matter what the experience was that caused them. Maybe I will let myself feel awful for a few hours, maybe a day. If the catalyst is severe (read: death of, harm to, or an illness of someone I love), maybe I will let myself stew for two days, but that is pretty much always the end of it, because I am in the driver's seat. I make the choices about how I feel, and I don't want to feel like crap and stifle my life, productivity, my relationships/interactions with others, or my ability to function or feel HAPPINESS for any longer than that.

Trust me when I tell you, I know what it's like to live through some pretty horrifying experiences. The kind of experiences that could easily allow someone to live in a state of depression forever.

You already know about the sudden death of my father and the chronic disease, but I've also experienced watching my sister slowly kill herself through heroin abuse, saw it rip my family apart over and over again (through various rehabs, her repeatedly stealing from all of us, her begging my parents to keep her locked up while she screamed and whaled going through withdrawal only to relapse again, wanting more than anything to see her get well, but truly not having any ability to do anything but love her when she would accept it) for over 26 years before she passed away in 2008 at the age of 43.

This was after supporting her through a liver transplant and everything that goes along with recovery from, and life after an organ transplantation procedure. Anyone who has loved (or still loves) someone who suffers from any addiction knows the toll that it can take on our lives. The love we feel for them, combined with the feeling of helplessness in our inabilities to do anything to truly help them get well is crippling. I stood next to my Mom on a windy October day, my arm around her as she tried to read the eulogy she had written without completely breaking down.

Death is something that our family has experienced often. In May of 2000, I stood in front of a large crowd and read the eulogy my mom had written for my aunt's funeral, just a few weeks before I graduated high school. My aunt, my mom's sister and best friend who we lived next door to for years, had fallen victim to cancer after fighting an incredibly brave battle for over ten years. My uncle on my dad's side passed away suddenly in 2007. Our family grew smaller and smaller. My faith in my ability to live a long life was tested time and time again. Three months ago, my last living uncle died of cancer very quickly over a six-month period. I have grown an emotional callus to death over the course of my life, although it never gets any easier to comprehend the fact that you will never have the chance to speak to or be in the presence of that person again.

In 2008, I was informed after a routine gynecological exam that I had cancerous cells on my cervix, and that I would need to go through several surgical procedures to *hopefully* eradicate those cells. What? Where the F did that come from? The level of simply not knowing what to expect, not knowing if I would be able to get rid of these cells, not knowing if full-blown cervical cancer would be the next medical issue I had to weather was debilitating at first.

The fact that various aunts and uncles (from both my mom's and dad's side) died from various forms of cancer wasn't all that reassuring, either, during this time period. But by that time, I already had my training. I already had the tools to choose my emotional state. So I used them. I said that no matter what, even if cervical cancer was the result, I would CHOOSE to be happy. Hell, if I was going to possibly die much sooner than expected, I wasn't going to waste what precious time I had left feeling bad for myself.

In fact, I was going to be better to myself than I had ever been before. Treat my body with the respect it deserved. Exercise, yoga, vegetables. If nothing else, I was committed to creating a clean internal environment that cancer would have a hard time replicating in. I had the surgeries, and still we waited. We had to wait because the only way to know if it worked was to wait, be re-tested in three months, six months, nine months, one year after the procedures. All that time waiting, not knowing if the cells were in there replicating and growing or dying off. But still, I practiced being happy, using my body as the main tool to produce those feelings.

I also read a variety of books on the subject of reversing cancer through nutrition and physical fitness. I stopped eating meat (which I have since picked back up, but much less frequently) and loaded up on vegetables, fruits, nuts, seeds, and beans, and also drank tons of water. At the end of the day, who really knows what caused the end result of the cells being eradicated (and staying away for the past seven years)? But I do know this: choosing to be happy and to love and honor my mind and body through the process were the right choices for me.

Here is the final, most powerful tool that we as human beings have to choose our emotional state: get grateful. Choose gratitude. Here is what I mean and how to actually put this into practice. I believe with every fiber of my being that gratitude trumps all other emotions. That if we consciously choose to feel gratitude, nothing else can fully exist in its presence. Not anger, not fear, not sadness, not frustration or any other negative emotion that we as humans naturally want to move away from feeling on any regular basis.

I also know that every single person in this world has a large variety of things to be grateful for, even if those things are not abundantly clear immediately. First and foremost for me are the people in my life, both past and present, and all they have taught me.

I am eternally grateful for every second I got to spend with my dad before he passed away, because even though I was a child, the life lessons he taught me stood the test of time. He taught me that you don't have to be the smartest or the strongest, only the hardest working, that life is meant to be enjoyed, and that a sense of humor is invaluable.

I am endlessly grateful for my mom, for every single thing she has ever taught me and will continue to teach me. For showing me what it looks like to stand strong in the face of adversity with grace and a peaceful heart, even when everything in your life is crumbling down around you. For the unconditional love and support she has shown and continues to show me, even when I was a total bitch to her and pushed her away throughout my tumultuous teenage years. For leading by example regarding how to treat other people, by showing me that treating others with love, respect, and kindness no matter what kind of mood we are in or what is going on in our lives not only benefits them and could be the difference maker in someone else's day, but also in our own.

I am grateful for my husband for accepting all of me, all of my strengths and all of my flaws, and loving me no matter what. For always following his passions with indescribable drive, encouraging me to do the same, and supporting me through it all. For allowing me to grow and change, and growing and changing along with me, even when neither of us is sure of the terrain ahead on the chosen path. For never saying that anything is impossible.

I am grateful for my best friend, Alexis, who is truly my family and has been a part of my life since we were six years old. For learning and growing and laughing uncontrollably together through incredible happiness, and for supporting each other through unimaginable loss and sadness. For speaking a language that only she and I understand.

I am grateful for every pet I've ever had, and for nature in general, and our incredible planet Earth. I am grateful for walks in the park, feeling the sun on my face, and the wind in my hair. I am grateful that I have a roof over my head and clean water running out of my faucets. I am grateful that I have heat in the winter and air conditioning in the summer. I am grateful that I have the power of free will. I am grateful that diabetes has taught me so many valuable life lessons, and that I was able to change my mind about what diabetes means to me, and the relationship I have with it each day. I am grateful for technological advances in medicine, in communication, in all forms. I am grateful to be alive here and now.

Now it's your turn. What I just did above is an incredibly powerful technique called "gratitude stacking." What that means is taking a few minutes to sit quietly (eyes closed, breathing deeply, hand over heart) and list all the things for which we are grateful and why. One thing after the next, only stopping when we truly cannot think of anything else. There is nothing–no person or experience–too small to be grateful for.

If you choose to practice this technique daily, especially when feeling negative emotions, not only will your mood change immediately in the moment, but allowing ourselves to feel intense gratitude at any time causes real physiological and hormonal changes in our bodies, the effects of which lasting for hours after we've finished the exercise. Gratitude is like healing medicine for the mind, body, and soul. And just like exercise, the more often we do it, the stronger our gratitude muscle becomes, and the easier it is to flex any time we need it. We never run the risk of practicing gratitude too much or too often…the more frequently we practice, the better off we will be.

ACTION ITEM–GRATITUDE STACKING: Before you do this action item, write down the 1-3 emotions you are feeling most strongly at this very moment, or that you have been feeling most strongly today. After you've written them down, take five minutes right now (put the book down, set a timer on your cellphone) and practice gratitude stacking. It's okay if you can't think of a myriad of things right away, or maybe you will find that five minutes just isn't enough time to list all of the things for which you are grateful. Either way, don't give up or stop trying.

If you don't have a lot of people in your life for whom you are grateful, move on to experiences you have had, and to other things that we often take for granted, like getting to go to grade school, high school, and/or college, and having running water, food, and shelter. Get creative and let your mind search for things to be grateful for. You might be surprised with what comes out of your own brain, and you might even cry (I do almost every time), which is a natural reaction to feeling intense gratitude and appreciation.

When the five minutes are up, immediately write down the top 1-3 emotions you are feeling at that moment. Compare them to the ones you wrote down before the exercise, and see how they have changed. I feel confident that this five-minute exercise (that we can do anytime, anywhere) will have a powerful effect on your emotional state. It is my hope that you will use this tool often in order to exercise your power of choice when it comes to the emotional state of mind we live in day-to-day.

Physiology: Believe it or not, the most immediate way to change the way we are feeling at any given moment is through physical movement, because the very act of changing our physiology in itself changes our focus. Movement of the physical body in any way, whether it be taking a brisk walk, doing jumping jacks, doing a plank right there on the floor, doing squats into our office chair, or any other short burst of energy will change our mental attitude and our focus every time. This works especially well when we consciously think about the fact that we are changing our physiology to improve our current psychology.

ACTION ITEM: Try this out right away. Rate the level of energy and enthusiasm that it takes you to get started (or continue on with) whatever tasks your day consists of. Rate yourself at a one if you can barely get yourself out of bed to use the bathroom, and a ten if you are bursting at the seams with energy, ready for anything! Get up and do 30 seconds to five minutes of physical movement in any form (jumping jacks, squats, high-knees, sit ups, planks, etc.), with the directed focus and intention of learning a lesson if there is something specific bothering you, or just have the simple intention of immediately moving forward in your day with a better attitude.

Very often, the only thing standing between our mental state and our success in keeping our attitude and focus on making progress in any situation is our willingness to MOVE, and again, the willingness to take the ACTION to correct our focus. Be sure to rate yourself on the same scale as soon as you are done to see how much more energized you really feel. Use this scale as many times throughout the day as you need to, in order to keep your mood and energy level where you want them to be.

One other tool that has been a hugely effective, instant mood-changer, not only in my life but in the lives of hundreds of thousands of others, is a mini-trampoline, also known as a rebounder. Yes, I'm serious! You can get one from $50, all the way up past $300 on *Amazon* and other online retailers (they do have weight limits, so be sure to read the details), and they are a game-changer when it comes to changing our physiology. We have one in the corner of our living room in between the couch and the wall (there is not much extra space here but we make it work), and both my husband and I use it every single morning.

The simple act of bouncing up and down (this doesn't have to be jumping; your feet don't even have to leave the surface) changes the physiology of our minds and bodies. It also has other added benefits, like helping our lymphatic system cleanse itself more efficiently, and, in general, it's just fun. Five to ten minutes of light bouncing to your favorite station on *Pandora* is an incredibly powerful way to change your emotional state.

The one we use at home is made by JumpSport, but there are other totally effective, less expensive versions as well. Be aware of the weight limits, as all makes and models are not necessarily the same. Another great free resource for physiology-changing exercises and explanations of the proper form in which to do them l is my *YouTube* channel, **https://www.youtube.com/user/824daniele,** which contains a variety of free videos showing how we can quickly and properly exercise anytime anywhere, regardless of whether we have any equipment or not (much more to come on that later)!

The bottom line is this: we can't control diabetes, but we can control the actions we take and the decisions we make about our diabetes care. Moving our bodies is one of the most important choices we have to make for the wellness of both our blood sugars and our mindsets!

Language/Questions/Thoughts: The way we feel, particularly the thoughts we focus on most, are heavily influenced by the language we use and the questions we ask most often in our everyday life. When we decide to accomplish something new in our lives, like creating a new habit, something we have wanted for a long time but have never been able to achieve before, our words make all the difference in whether we succeed or succumb to self-sabotage. And self-sabotage gets its fuel from our thoughts and our language. Notice that I don't say "fail," because even when we try and don't reach the exact outcome we set out for, it is still a success as long as we objectively reassess, make some changes, and try again.

The words we choose to use and the questions we choose to ask ourselves throughout the process of forming new habits are crucial. Logically speaking, if we always say things like "I suck at this" or "I'm not good at this" or "this is too hard," or ask questions like "why me?" "why do bad things always happen to me?", or say things like "I have such bad luck" or "FML" or "why can't I ever catch a break?" we will find that we will have a much tougher time reaching our goals. These words and phrases presuppose that all of these things are true, and our brains believe what we tell them.

I know all too well that we're all our own worst critics. That can be a good thing if we learn how to take a step back when things don't go the way we planned and allow our shortcomings to teach us how to proceed better the next time around. However, it can also be a very bad thing if we choose to talk to ourselves disrespectfully, or in a way that cuts us down or diminishes our self-worth, since that kind of self-talk suffocates progress, motivation, and inspiration.

The language I used to use throughout the extensive internal dialogue during my teenage years was atrocious. I would berate myself, not only for being overweight, but for every bit of food I ate and for every blood sugar I saw that was out of range, and that was pretty much every single day. The names I would call myself make me sick to think about now. The thought of talking to anyone with that level of disrespect, let alone myself, makes me cringe and want to go back and give my teenage self a huge hug and tell her that things will eventually be okay.

I used to tell myself all the time that I was cursed. That I must have been a mass murderer in a previous life, carrying some serious bad karma, and that I obviously deserved all the pain and suffering I was experiencing. I told myself that so many times, pretty much every time something went wrong, and it became part of my story, part of my belief system, all because I said it enough times that it became true for me. It also gave me an easy out, an easy answer for my brain to accept when other things went wrong.

At least I knew it was because I deserved to be miserable because of something I did somewhere else, long ago, on another plane of existence. That was my language, my belief, and my reality. I was miserable and depressed because I deserved to be. That language and belief allowed me to numb my brain to doing any real work to figure out how to make things better for myself. If I deserved it, then it was just meant to be, no other questions needed to be asked. Right? That's what I thought until I began asking myself a whole new set of questions.

The human brain is just plain magical. So magical that even today, with the incredible technology we have and the genius minds that are working on it, we still have barely begun to understand the true capacities and abilities that the human brain possesses. However, there are certain aspects of the brain that we do understand, and one of the simplest things our brains do automatically is that when asked a question, they immediately begin to look for answers, particularly answers to support the tonality and contextual ques in the question.

The answers our brains come up with are directly affected by the quality of the questions we ask them. This is where the action comes into play. This is where we need to come up with some new, productive questions to replace our old, unproductive questions so that we can really put our brains to work for us instead of against us.

ACTION ITEM: Examining the questions we ask ourselves on a regular basis is crucial to changing our habits and achieving our goals. Write down three questions that you know you ask yourself on a regular basis. Questions that prompt our brains to look for answers that presuppose the circumstances in the question, and that support the quality of the question asked. Here are some common examples that many clients have shared with me over the years, and that I believe we have all asked ourselves more than once in the past.

Old Questions:

1. **Why do I have such bad luck?** This allows the brain to presuppose a couple of things. One, that we have bad luck without any room for doubt, making it easy to ignore all of the things that have happened in our lives that could easily be perceived as good luck; and two, that luck is even a real thing.
2. **Why do bad things always happen to me?** This allows the brain to presuppose that bad things always happen to us, making it easy to forget all of the good things in our lives and all of the reasons we have to be grateful.

3. **Why can't I catch a break?** This allows the brain to presuppose that not only can't we catch whatever it is that each of us individually perceives to be a break, but it also prompts the brain not to search out all of the examples of times in our lives that we very well may have caught our own definition of a break.

New Questions:

1. What lesson(s) can I learn from this experience?
2. What values or beliefs can I fortify in my life from this experience?
3. How can I take what could easily be perceived as a negative experience and instead, find a valuable lesson to inspire myself and others in the future when unexpected conditions come up?
4. What action(s) could I take differently next time in order to achieve a different result?

What are your old, comfortable, go-to questions? What are your new, productive, resourceful questions? All of the new questions prompt our brains to come up with real, viable answers that will help us move forward after experiencing any situation that would normally send us down the road of unproductive questions. Getting our thoughts out into a journal with a pen and paper, or an online journal, is an incredibly powerful exercise that we can use any time to direct our thoughts and the language we use with ourselves and others.

It might be slow-going at first, or your brain might just start pouring out incredible suggestions right from the start…you never know unless you ask! And after practicing this for a while, eventually we find that we are now asking more productive questions and choosing our thoughts and focuses more automatically, more habitually. This allows us to be in better moods more often, and just feel calmer and less overwhelmed by life in general.

Animal Videos, Breaking our Patterns, and Changing our Emotional States

Like most of the world, I enjoy a cute animal video from time to time. Kittens, puppies, baby birds, you name it, I love them all. Animal videos have some of the highest viewer ratings of any category of videos on the internet, across all countries and continents. Why is that? Have you ever been with another person while watching one of these videos? Seen the way both your and the other person's facial expressions change? How body language changes, mood changes? How more often than not, we want to watch another one right away?

What feelings and emotions are animal videos tapping into to alter our mental states that way? After years of studying human psychology, it's hard for me not to look a little deeper into any phenomenon that is so incredibly popular across all of humanity, and that visibly changes a person's mental state and attitude in such short order. Why is it that seeing warm, fuzzy kittens dozing off quite literally makes us feel–well–warm and fuzzy? There is some real science going on here!

I'm a big fan of using tools that are always accessible (and free) in order to take action to break a negative pattern and change our current negative emotional state into a more productive, resourceful state of mind. When we are feeling unpleasant emotions, it is very often due to habitual patterns which we run through in our minds on a regular basis. Take checking our blood sugar, for example, something most of us do many times every day. When I check my blood sugar, it's too easy to be affected in some way by the number on the meter. There was a long period of time in my life where every time I checked my blood sugar and it was over 150, I would immediately begin to ask myself what I did wrong, why I couldn't get things right (super unproductive questions), and even insult myself for not being in range.

And after having the pleasure of working with and becoming close friends with so many people who live with diabetes, I found out that I am not the only person who can very easily slip into a negative pattern and emotional state based off a blood sugar reading. We have these patterns for everything we experience in life, and the only way to break an old pattern is to continually interrupt it as soon as we recognize that it's happening, and introduce a new pattern.

ACTION ITEM: Pick a pattern that you know you run regularly in your own life. Maybe it's the insulting yourself after checking your blood sugar pattern that I used to run. Maybe it's the overeating because of boredom pattern. Maybe it's the putting yourself down for skipping exercise pattern (I used to run all of these patterns in my daily life). The next time you catch yourself starting to fall into that old pattern, consciously choose to use your more productive questions from the previous action item, and then follow-up those questions with a minute or two of animal videos. I know it might sound funny or ridiculous, but the fact stands that we release endorphins when we see something that makes us happy, so why not use an animal video as a tool to change our current mindset? First, ask some productive questions to get your brain working, then let the endorphins kick in, and get back to reaching your goals.

The only bad side to cute animal videos is that because they make us so happy, it's easy to get sucked in and spend too much time watching. Try to limit the mood-altering videos to a five-minute maximum, then back to focus, goal-setting and taking action.

Self-Sabotage, Feeling Overwhelmed, Failure, and Fear: These terms, although not pleasant to deal with, are all very real phenomena that, if we don't consistently address every time we set new goals for ourselves, will always end up getting the best of us. Self-sabotage is one of the worst things we can do to ourselves, yet also the most common. We are really good at getting in our own way when trying to make any kind of progress.

For example, have you ever said on a Friday that you are going to start eating healthy on Monday, then proceed to gorge the whole weekend in preparation for the new healthy eating plan? I've done that exact thing more than once, and I know that the majority of people have had the same experience. And in the moment, we mean it. We really want to commit to a new nutrition plan on Monday, we really do want to provide our bodies with the healthy foods it needs to give us the energy we need to best support our lives.

The challenge is that we didn't, right then at that moment (or beforehand), plan out and shop for our meals for the upcoming week. Maybe we went the route of planning the first few days because we were following some sort of cleanse, and committed to eating only lettuce and lemons or something like that. And maybe we did that for a day or two or three, but in either scenario, by the third or fourth day, we were finding it much more difficult to stay on track, and by nightfall were eating something unhealthy. This is self-sabotage.

One, we didn't plan the entire week from start to finish, we failed to plan and therefore planned to fail. Two, we may have also committed to something extremely restrictive and unrealistic that would provide unhealthy, unsustainable results if followed for too long. Back in my years of depression and binge-eating, I believed that the ten minutes it would take me to plan out my meals for the week and the hour to shop for them were less important than watching the next episode of the *X-Files*. Needless to say, my blood sugars and my physical body reflected my priorities and my beliefs.

Where your focus goes, your energy flows. Such a simple statement, but at the same time, so incredibly powerful. I was focused on TV, not on making a list of groceries and meals I wanted to eat for the upcoming week, so that's where my energy flowed...into the TV. Whatever we train our minds to focus on (our dominating thoughts), that's what we will get more of.

Mitigating self-sabotage starts with five minutes of planning ahead. Try it out. If you put as much or more focus on meal preparation, water intake, and checking your blood sugar than you do on watching TV, surfing the internet and all of its social media or video-sharing sites, gaming, and/or whatever it is you focus on more than your health, you will automatically get better results because you are consciously changing your actions. And the best part is that you can decide to focus your thoughts on whatever you choose.

Take it slow, don't put too much on your proverbial plate. Plan out one day ahead of time, then execute. Then plan out three days in advance, and execute. Don't move on to the next level until you have gotten a handle on things. Work your way up to a week. Slowly become okay with the fact that things might not go as planned all the time, and when things do go wrong, don't let that be a reason to stray from the plan you set out for yourself. Expect the unexpected and roll with the punches as you build new habits.

It is impossible to make major changes to our health and habits without feeling overwhelmed. Feeling overwhelmed is a natural reaction to changing our actions and breaking old, worn-in patterns. Think of overwhelming feelings as a signal our bodies send us to let us know that change is occurring. Change really does happen outside of our comfort zones, and it's easy to feel overwhelmed when we are uncomfortable.

The most successful people in life are those who are willing to be uncomfortable in order to reach the next level, no matter what the endeavor. It was overwhelming for my body to adjust while I was in the process of losing over 65 pounds. Because my blood sugars ran so high for so long, I reached a point where I was feeling the signs of low blood sugar when my blood sugar was around 100-120. This was a real problem for a while, since 80-120 was my blood sugar target range, yet I was feeling unable to function normally in that range. It was overwhelming to say the least.

I gave up on working hard on it many times, allowing it to return to the back burner, even though I knew it was one of the most important aspects of my diabetes management. My body needed time to reset itself to a new normal, but back then, I didn't know nearly as much about the human body's incredible ability to change and adapt and support our goals. Eventually, after slowly bringing my A1c down from 13+%, my body began to adjust to the new normal. Today, I feel the signs of low blood sugar when I'm around 70 or so, allowing me to function normally in my target range.

This didn't happen overnight. It didn't even happen in a week, and back then, I didn't know if it would ever happen for sure. But I knew it was something I wanted and needed. And it did eventually happen after I understood, accepted, and embraced the fact that feeling overwhelmed is and always will be part of the equation when trying to make sustainable health changes. And eventually, we reach the next level. One where the actions that once made us feel overwhelmed now feel like the new normal. When we expect feelings and emotions to arise, it is easier to deal with them when they come up, and continue to move forward. Expect to be overwhelmed, and embrace it as a part of making changes.

The last part of the Mindset section discusses the two "F" words that hold humanity back from making progress more than anything else in history, the "F" words that everyone hates the most. Failure and fear…and fear of failure. These two words have the ability to hold so much power over us, our mindsets, and the paths, risks, and chances we choose to take if we let them. First, let's talk about failure.

Failure is inevitable, expected, and a major component of making real, sustainable changes in our lives. Failure has the ability to teach us life lessons, and to shape our awareness so that we know, moving forward, what does and what does not work. Without failure, we would have no life experience, and without life experience, we would not have the ability to learn lessons and help others through our experiences. Failure is a gift; we have just been so conditioned to see it instead as shameful, as a downfall, a reason to give up on our goals, a reason to feel less than enough. I believe that failure is inherently necessary on the road to success.

Failure builds character and strength of will. Failure allows us to be humble (we are all only human) and also to be more intelligent when we make our next move. The biggest problem with failure is that in the moment, it sucks, there's no denying that. It has the ability to make us feel negative emotions when we realize we have failed at an attempt to accomplish something. But just like any other situation in life that doesn't go according to plan (this equates to mostly all situations in my life), it is our reaction to it, our attitude towards it that shapes the reality we experience.

What if we all saw failure as a gift to be appreciated, a gift we need to open to propel us forward? What if we all experienced failure merely as a temporary setback that we needed in order to get to the next level? The key is allowing failure to humble us, to strengthen us, to teach us, to shape our next moves. The key is not allowing failure to hold us down, not allowing it to be the reason we feel bad about ourselves, not allowing failure to keep us stagnant and defeated.

We have a very real choice when it comes to failure: we can either let it defeat us, or let it fortify us. We can even let it do some combination of the two. However, the most important factor involved when we experience failure is whether or not we pick ourselves up, dust ourselves off, acknowledge where things went wrong, make a few adjustments, and keep moving forward and making progress towards our goals. Failure is valuable life experience that we all need, whether we realize it or not.

There is not enough room in this book for me to recount all of the failures I've experienced throughout my life, some more life-altering than others. There is no human being who has ever accomplished any meaningful goal they have set for themselves without failing (often many times). No person is exempt from failure. I like to think logically, and logic dictates that when we set out to reach a goal, we should factor in a plan for mitigating the suck-factor of failure. We need to have a plan of action ready to put into play so that failure no longer puts us down for the count, but instead fuels us to get back up and fight harder (and smarter) than before.

And then there is fear. Fear is an emotion that, more than any other, keeps us from taking action, making changes, reaching goals, and being truly happy. Fear of failure (although we now know failure is nothing to fear), fear of looking stupid, fear of what other people will think of us, fear of not being enough, fear of not being loved and accepted. These are some of the top things of which we as humans are fearful, and when we get caught up in thinking about them over and over again (where your focus goes, your energy flows), we're stopped dead in our tracks. These fears stop us from taking the actions we need to take in order to finally lose that excess body fat for good, stop us from exercising because we fear having low blood sugars, stop us from starting a new relationship because we are afraid of what the other person will think about our diabetes, stop us from (fill in the blank with what fear stops you from doing most often).

Fear is something we struggle with, the thing that, once we take two steps forward, often makes us take one step back. Instead, we are best-served to dance with fear rather than struggling against it. We can't stop feeling fear, but we can change the way we react when it pops up in our lives.

Fear is like an automatically regulated thermostat. When we set an automatic thermostat at 72 degrees Fahrenheit, as soon as the temperature starts rising or falling, the automatic component kicks in to heat up or cool down the room, with the aim of getting back to the set temperature. The problem is that our willingness to act in the face of fear is also regulated much in the same way. We all have our own comfort levels, the zones in which we feel most able to function. And when we become fearful of something, our bodies and minds do everything they can to bring us back to that pre-set comfort zone so we don't feel that fear anymore. Therein lies a huge challenge.

When we set out to change our health, to change our choices around our diabetes management, it's scary. We are used to the level we have been operating on, so when we start turning up the heat and feeling the fear associated with the possibility of getting burned (read: failure), it's natural to want to bring things back down to that previous comfort level. The way to use fear to our advantage is to intentionally set a new "comfort zone," a new temperature, that becomes our normal operating conditions. That way, we can immediately recognize fear when it rears its ugly head.

We can say, "Hey fear, I know that's you trying to automatically regulate me back to my old comfort zone, but I'm creating a new comfort zone, and you are not needed here. I'm no longer operating on auto-pilot, I'm in control and I know what I'm doing." Maybe that sounds silly to you, but don't knock it till you try it. Just becoming aware of failure and fear in these different contexts could be the thing that helps you stay on track. When we change our awareness about anything, it automatically changes the decisions we make around that topic, simply due to having more extensive knowledge than we had before. As Franklin D. Roosevelt so accurately put it, "The only thing we have to fear is fear itself."

Change – Understand, Accept, and Embrace that Change is the Price of Survival

When I was in my late teens, and even through my mid-20s, my focus was hazy at best. I went from this job to that job, always doing well, but never really focusing on any one thing. I was a bartender, a waitress, a chef, an office manager, a realtor. All of these were jobs where I worked with people to get them a result they were after, whether it was a gin and tonic or a three-story townhouse. But, as the years went on, I never really felt satisfied or fulfilled with my work at the end of the day.

Even though I was working with people, which is one of my true passions, I wasn't serving them in a way that allowed me to add the maximum value to their lives; therefore, I wasn't feeling the maximum value in my life. I also wasn't fully focused on my health. My health was not yet my number one priority in life at this point, either. By my mid-20s, I wasn't completely out of control anymore, but I wasn't CONSISTENTLY taking the actions needed in order to dominate my diabetes, either.

I was still occasionally visiting my own pity-party, still blaming diabetes for my unhappiness when it suited me. I was getting more and more mentally restless by the day, but just couldn't figure out what my next step should be. Little did I know that diabetes, the thing I blamed most for my unhappiness, would end up being the vehicle I would use to share my genuine passion for serving others. It was at that point in my life that I was led to an event where I realized that diabetes didn't happen TO me, it happened FOR me, and that was a life-changing moment.

Have you ever heard the saying, "When the student is ready, the teacher will appear"? The chain of events that took place next in my life, and the choices I made based on those events truly shaped my destiny, and allowed me to discover my other true passion in life, by allowing me to unlock my love of health, fitness, and nutrition, of which only glimmers had been peeking through before. Learning and embodying the skills I needed to continually improve my health, and then feeling compelled to share my years of experiences in the realm of diabetes management, fat loss, muscle building, and body re-composition didn't just happen as I passively sat by.

I had to take actions that I never had before (that I never thought I was capable of) in order to get this new result. This chain of events couldn't have come as more of an unexpected surprise, something that, had you asked me about it the day before, I would have laughed in skepticism. Something that if I had not become laser-focused on, would most likely not have come to the beautiful fruition that it has at this point, allowing me to do what I love every single day and call it my career.

> *"Love what you do and do what you love. Don't listen to anyone else who tells you not to do it."*
> – Ray Bradbury

That is one thing I can say is true, without a shadow of a doubt, in order to experience the ultimate happiness in your life. The fulfillment I feel when I am able to add value to someone's life, to serve them, to empower them, to help them build their health and confidence is something that is difficult to describe in words. I believe all human beings experience fulfillment when we are able to be of service to others; however, being of service to others wasn't always something that I was focused on. The following is how I went from being a real estate agent who dreaded the routine and hated her job to who I am now, loving my work and feeling blessed every day to get to do what I do.

One morning while in our weekly staff meeting at the real estate office, our broker brought in a speaker to talk to us about boosting sales through different methods of connecting with people on a genuine level, and also by examining what we personally could be doing differently to better assist (serve) our clients. About 15 realtors sat around the conference room table eating bagels and drinking coffee when Christian came walking in. Let's just say he looked very well put-together, dressed nicely, was obviously physically fit, and noticeably confident.

Let me preface this with some background info about me and my personality at that point in my life. To call me a skeptical person would have been an understatement. If you were a salesman of any kind, I was your worst nightmare. When I wanted to buy anything at all, I did my research ahead of time and came in knowing exactly what I wanted, and was blatantly unwilling to listen to any BS sales pitch. You certainly weren't getting anything by on me, and I had my defenses up.

Christian then proceeded with his presentation. It was captivating, interactive, and inspiring. It touched on a deeply human element that I wasn't expecting. I was truly affected and moved by the valuable information he passed on to us, more so than in any other weekly meeting before, or in fact, in almost any presentation that I had seen in any capacity before in my life.

I learned quite a bit about myself and how I interacted with my clients (and other people in general), as well as new strategies that I could begin applying to my career immediately. To say that I was impressed would be an understatement. There was nothing sales-y about it, no tagline or reference to a product or service the entire time. So imagine my surprise when, at the end of Christian's 45-minute-long animated presentation, I learned that he did in fact have something to sell, and I wasn't immediately opposed to hearing about whatever it was.

Here is where it really gets weird. He was selling tickets to a seminar/live event called "Unleash the Power Within," or UPW for short, something I had never heard of before. It is a four-day seminar that runs from morning to night–total immersion, they call it–which would potentially help boost our sales and help us make overall improvements in the quality of our lives. And even though the first thought that entered my head was, "This is probably total BS," since that was, up until that point, how I reacted to anyone trying to sell me anything, I couldn't escape the incessant thoughts that were flying through my mind about how I felt after that presentation. It really felt like something inside me that was lying dormant was suddenly awake, and demanding attention.

If what I learned at the event was anything like what I learned in the previous 45 minutes, it could really be a life-changing experience, full of information that could help improve my career, I thought. I then did what up until that point in my life was unthinkable to me. I called my husband from the real estate office to let him know first, that I was going away to a four-day seminar (I welcomed him to join me; he politely declined and ended up going with me when I went again, for a second time, a year later, and he absolutely loved it), and second, I was going to pay for it–all $500 of it (not including hotel/travel) –on my credit card.

Now mind you, this was so far from my realm of normal activity that my husband wouldn't have been out of line if he asked who I was and what I did with his wife. However, taking that step so far outside of my comfort zone caused me to grow in ways I never imagined possible. Change really does happen outside of your comfort zone, you just have to be willing to follow your intuition, your gut, that voice inside your head that tells you to follow your instincts. And when you do, the results will continually amaze you, especially when it comes to your health.

Long story short, I entered that four-day live event (by myself) as a realtor who wanted to improve her sales and create meaningful relationships with clients, and I came out understanding more about myself, about who I really was, about my beliefs and values in life, what my priorities in life had been so far, and also that I was not at all interested in being a realtor anymore. I understood that I had been letting my fears, and my intense need to feel in control of everything all the time guide my decisions, and I also knew what I needed to do to deal with those limiting emotions to take my life to the next level. During those four days, I realized that in order for me to be truly happy and fulfilled with my life, I would first have to become truly happy and fulfilled with my HEALTH, which is the foundation for all human happiness.

Health is the ultimate foundation of all things, happiness included, and I just couldn't see that clearly before I went to this event, met some mentors and coaches, and was shown some tools to use to identify what areas of my life needed improvement and why. When I returned home that Sunday, I was a different person, and not just temporarily. I was laser-focused on the GOALS I had set for myself in the past four days, specifically getting my A1c below 7% on a consistent basis, eating only whole, real foods and cutting out all the take-out and chemical-laden processed, boxed foods I depended on daily, creating and sticking to a viable weekly workout plan for the upcoming three months, and reducing my insulin levels to support my new healthy-eating lifestyle.

For whatever reason, these were the things that were all of a sudden so incredibly important to me that I couldn't not do the things that would get me there; whereas before, I knew I should be doing these things, but they weren't a constant, pressing need. As you are probably already aware, knowing is not enough; we must fortify that knowledge with action. We all KNOW we should be eating healthy and exercising regularly for optimal blood sugar control and health, but many of us are not DOING these things, even though we are 100% acutely aware of their importance, and maybe already greatly suffering because we don't do them consistently. Something major inside me shifted during those four days in 2008, and life was never going to be the same again.

The bottom line and the point to this story is that in order to master the psychology of success, to embrace the Diabetes Dominator mentality, or really to achieve any goal in life, we need first to fully identify where we are right now, and how we got there in the first place. After years of thinking I had my priorities in order, I finally came to understand, after years of not realizing it, that health is the foundation for all human happiness. The sooner you embrace this reality, the sooner you will be on your way to feeling (and looking) the best you ever have, keeping it that way for the rest of your life, and ultimately paying it forward to your family, friends, and loved ones.

I assume (and hope!) the majority of us brush our teeth every day. We do this automatically upon waking because we have conditioned ourselves to believe that it is simply unacceptable not to, that it is a vital aspect of setting our day up right. Brushing our teeth is a choice, a habit, just like any other. And just like we brush our teeth every day, conditioning our mindset for success every day is just as (if not more) important.

You know that feeling you have when you need to brush your teeth when you wake up? It feels like there is a film of grime covering them, shielding their potential brightness and clarity (not to mention the nasty breath). The same goes for your mindset, but unfortunately, most people never consider the importance of conditioning their mindsets so that they have a clean, clear, fresh, productive, resourceful outlook each day. By choosing to commit to performing these daily, weekly, monthly, and yearly mindset-related actions, you will essentially be cleaning off years of built-up grime that has been clouding your abilities to make real progress towards your health goals.

And the best part is, each time you take these actions, it will be like building a muscle–the more consistently you work it, the stronger it will get. Your mindset will get stronger and stronger each time, building on the last "mental workout." This mental strength will not only change your perspectives throughout every aspect of your life, but it will also give you the tools by building the sustainable habits you need to stay on track and make the progress in your health that you have always wanted but were never able to fully realize and make a part of your everyday life.

13

NUTRITION

"Let food be thy medicine, and medicine be thy food."
-Hippocrates

Nutrition Basics – Nutrient Density and Whole Foods

Let's get into the food basics. The facts that allow us to make intelligent decisions about what we eat and how we fuel our one and only body that, for some reason, aren't a part of our basic education (this has always boggled my mind). Providing our bodies with the nutrition they need is by far one of the most important and beneficial life skills to have, since what we put into our bodies as fuel directly affects every aspect of our lives. These include our energy levels, mood, cognitive clarity (read: brain fog), blood sugar levels, weight, skin, hair, and nails. Other than drinking water (the most important aspect of living healthy), the foods we choose to eat determine the quality of our health and the quality of our lives.

There is so much information available today about so many different diets and nutrition lifestyles that I know it can get confusing and overwhelming. That is why we are going to cover Nutrition 101, so we can focus on learning some simple science that holds true for everyone, no matter what diet you choose. Treat it like a crash course for a test in college: once you learn and understand the basics, you will be able to pass the nutritional tests of life.

Learning and implementing this information also allows us to build a healthy-eating lifestyle that works for each of our own individual likes and goals. I am not going to promote any particular diet, as I believe that different nutritional lifestyles work well for different people. The two things I am going to promote heavily are nutrient density and whole foods. These are the two most important aspects to take into consideration when it comes to choosing the foods we eat on a regular basis. We will get more into what those things are and why they are so incredibly important in just a minute.

But first…**WATER.**

Other than oxygen, water is THE MOST ESSENTIAL thing that is vital to our bodies in order to sustain our health. I truly cannot stress enough how crucial being properly hydrated is to every single system that the human body contains. I could talk about it all day, every day because it is genuinely THAT IMPORTANT.

We have 11 major systems that are constantly doing their thing inside of us, most of them requiring no effort from us–they just happen naturally. Simply put, these are different systems within the body that work independently and together to form a properly functioning human body. I'm talking about our cardiovascular system that allows our lungs to breathe air–a person takes an average of 20,000 breaths each day, all without ever giving it much thought or effort. I'm talking about our circulatory system, which allows our hearts to pump on average 100,000 times per day without us even asking it to. Then there are our digestive systems, our reproductive systems, our lymph systems, and the list goes on and on.

My whole point of mentioning all of that is to try to emphasize that the human body is incredibly amazing and incredibly resilient. **It does all of these mind-blowing things for us every second of every day, and all it really wants in return, more than anything else, is enough water to do its jobs.** Water is the main fuel source for all of these systems to keep doing what they do. When we are dehydrated, these systems function much less optimally, and at certain levels of dehydration, begin to shut down completely. That is why it is so incredibly, majorly, vitally, crucially important to make drinking enough water every single day a top priority if we are on the journey to building a healthy lifestyle…there is simply nothing that takes higher precedence.

So how much water is enough? It's a super simple equation that works for everyone. One half of our body weight in ounces is the minimum amount required for keeping our body systems happily fueled and functioning optimally. You weigh 200 pounds? 100 ounces of water per day, minimum. We also need more water as we lose it, meaning through sweating, or even less appealing avenues such as vomiting or diarrhea.

The best way to keep track of how much water you're drinking in a day is to get a reusable water bottle and figure out how many times in a day you must fill it up in order to reach your water needs...and just do it, starting first thing in the morning as soon as you open your eyes. Fill your water bottle before you go to bed, keep it on the nightstand, and consciously decide to drink water first thing upon waking. Before you go to the bathroom, before you check your phone, before you do anything, drink as much of that water as you comfortably can. That way, you are getting a jumpstart on your day, giving your body the fuel it needs to get you going, since you haven't hydrated at all throughout the night. Make this part of your morning routine, and the benefits to the rest of your day will be endless.

Now, if you are someone who barely drinks any water on a regular basis, or not much, you may need to slowly scale your water consumption up, adding however much water per day you are comfortable with until you reach your minimum requirement needs. Starting with one full water bottle, and adding 10-20 ounces per day is a good place to start, or you can just go for the whole thing, all depending on how you feel. If you are not used to drinking enough water, you will have to pee more often for the first couple of weeks to a month of finally getting enough water. This is your body's way of saying "thank you" for giving it the water it needs to flush out toxins that were being stored in fat cells. Once your body becomes used to the new normal of being properly hydrated and has had a chance to flush things out, the pee schedule will return to normal.

One more thing that I have heard many times over the years of working with and coaching so many people regarding healthy habits is that some people say they don't like the taste of water. Although I find it to be pretty tasteless, I like to make sure there are viable, healthy options for everyone to get their water in a way that is enjoyable. There are many ways to change the taste of water in a healthy way.

This includes adding any fruit, vegetable, or herb to your water. Filling a pitcher of water and adding a few slices of cucumber and a few sprigs of mint completely changes the flavor of the water. Another great addition is slicing up some strawberries and an orange and putting those in the pitcher. The flavor possibilities are only limited by the produce options at the store and your imagination.

There are also ways of changing the flavor of water that are not healthy. These unhealthy options include processed additives such as Crystal Light, Mio, or any other powdered or liquid additive that have a laundry list of unrecognizable chemicals on the ingredient label. Adding processed chemicals to our water is not a healthy way to hydrate and be kind to our bodies. Soda, juice, milk, Gatorade, or any other bottled or powdered beverage does not count towards reaching our daily water needs.

The only other thing that counts towards hydration is caffeine-free tea (hot or iced) that you make yourself at home by boiling…water! I talk about water so much because the level of importance it holds when it comes to human health is just so paramount. Staying properly hydrated consistently is the most important place to start when creating a healthy lifestyle, and it just so happens to be one of the easiest, most inexpensive things to actually implement. The action of getting hydrated is up to you! If there was ever a best place to get started on implementing new habits, choosing to drink plenty of water is it.

What is a whole food?

According to the incomparable, all-knowing Interweb, a whole food is any food that is unprocessed and unrefined, or processed and refined as little as possible, before being consumed. Whole foods do not contain preservatives or added ingredients of any kind. In my own loosest of definitions, whole foods can be broken down into five categories: vegetables, fruits, nuts, seeds, and beans. As far as needing the least amount of processing, or alteration to their original state before we eat them, all of these groups are as close to whole foods as it gets.

Meat and dairy, unless you are literally milking the cow and drinking the milk right then, or catching a fish and eating it sashimi style on the spot, is not going to be what I would consider a whole food. All meat and dairy must be processed in some way to get to our tables. Don't get me wrong, I do eat meat now and then, and on very rare occasion I will have dairy, but over the years, I have found that a whole foods, plant-based nutritional lifestyle works the best for me and my diabetes and weight management.

Plant-based doesn't necessarily mean that meat is out of the picture, it just means that things that have grown directly out of the earth are the bulk of my meals, and if I'm eating meat, it's just a guest at the plant-based party. Again, I can't stress enough that this is what works best for me, but might not be the best option for everyone. This is why we all must take the time to learn the basics so we can build the nutritional lifestyle that works best for each of us…one that properly nourishes our bodies and minds, and also makes us feel happy, satisfied, and successful.

At the simplest level (remember, just the basics here), everything we eat can essentially be placed into three categories, called macronutrients. Macronutrients are where calories come from. These macronutrients are carbohydrates, protein, and fat, all of which are listed on all nutrition labels, and all have healthy sources and unhealthy sources. By "sources," I mean the foods (or food-like substances) we consume to get these macronutrients into our bodies. The human body needs all three macronutrients to function optimally, and I never recommend completely cutting out any of them.

Check out my website, **diabetesdominator.com,** to download my healthy and unhealthy food lists that are great to use as guidelines for shopping lists when reading ingredient labels, as well as a pantry clean-out guide so you know what has to go in order to treat your body with the nutritional respect it deserves. For now, let's learn some simple math that will always remain constant so you never have to guess where your calories are coming from, then we will dive deeper into each of the three macronutrients.

Do you ever look at a nutrition label and see the calories in a serving of that item and wonder where the calories are coming from? Here is a simple way to always know what's what. Every calorie we ever eat comes from those three macronutrients (carbohydrates, proteins, and fats), and the formula for figuring out how many calories is coming from each macronutrient never changes. There are also calories that come from alcohol, which is a different category in itself (not a macronutrient!), and for the sake of reality (statistics say that the average American consumes four alcoholic beverages per week), I will include alcohol in here, too.

1 gram of carbs = 4 calories

1 gram of protein = 4 calories

1 gram of fat = 9 calories

1 gram of alcohol = 7 calories

That's it, 4, 4, 9, and sometimes 7. For example, if we look at a juice box that we use to correct lows, we might see that it has 15 grams of carbs in one serving, which is the whole juice box (depending on the brand and size). When we multiply 15 carbs by four calories, we find that the juice box contains 60 calories. It really is that simple. So the next time you are looking at a nutrition label and want to know how many calories are coming from carbs for example, just multiply the grams of carbs per serving by four, and you will have your answer. Same for protein: multiply the grams of protein per serving by four, and you will know how many calories are coming from protein. Lastly, multiply the grams of fat per serving by nine, and you will know how many calories are coming from fat.

There is no need to be confused by nutrition labels if you just focus on these three foundational factors. Of course, there are other factors involved beyond the three macronutrients, but first understanding how macronutrients and calories are related is very helpful. Calories come from macronutrients, it really is that simple. This multiplication trick is just a quick tool that I find helpful when I want to know what I'm getting into.

Before I go any further I have to share an incredibly crucial insight that I've learned the (very) hard way myself, and that I've seen so many clients struggle with over the years. One thing that I believe to be of paramount importance when it comes to changing our habits, to learning about and applying new nutrition information (or any information for that matter) to our lives is that perfection should never be what we are striving for. The most important thing to stay focused on is making progress–small, permanent changes, doing a little better today than we did yesterday. Striving for perfection is like constantly trying to capture a unicorn; it simply isn't possible, it will never happen.

Because perfection is an unattainable goal, striving for it becomes a vicious form of self-sabotage, because it gives us a reason to feel negatively about ourselves and our efforts ALL OF THE TIME, and gives us an excuse to give up more easily because we are never able to reach this imaginary level of

perfection, no matter how hard we try. I recommend throwing "perfect" out the window and running over it a few times to make sure it's gone, because it can too easily be the end of many valiant efforts to improve our health and wellness. Perfection is a killer of dreams, inspiration, and motivation. Don't let a unicorn control your ability to feel successful and proud of your efforts! If you are one of the many people who describe themselves as a perfectionist, (like I used to be) NOW is always the right time to do yourselves a huge favor and eradicate the term from your vocabulary.

ACTION ITEM: Go grab something from your kitchen that has a nutrition label on it and try out the 4, 4, 9 trick. Sometimes, even the nutrition labels aren't perfect, and that's okay. Try it out on something that has all three macronutrients in it (peanut butter, for example), and see if it all adds up. And if it isn't exact, it's okay, because nothing is perfect!

What is Nutrient Density?

Of all the nutritional terminology being used in the world today, I strongly believe that nutrient density is the most important one to understand, implement, and embrace. It is the key factor that truly has the biggest impact on our overall health and wellness when it comes to fueling our bodies with what they need. Simply stated, nutrient density means how many nutrients that are healthy for our bodies (that our bodies need, and are easy for our bodies to absorb and assimilate) that we get from a food per calorie it contains. Nutrient density is a simple way to connect nutrients with the amount of calories in our food.

For example, one cup of sliced strawberries contains about 50 calories (broken down into approximately 12 grams of carbs, one gram of protein, three grams of fiber, 26 milligrams of calcium, 255 milligrams of potassium, Vitamin A, Vitamin B, Vitamin C, Vitamin E, and Vitamin K, in addition to other minerals and phytochemicals, all of which are amazingly beneficial to our bodies), while one cup of strawberry jelly contains about 800 calories (208 grams of carbs, and no other nutrients AT ALL). It's the same one-cup measurement—heck, same fruit for that matter—but certainly not the same nutrient density. We could describe the sliced strawberries as "nutrient-dense," and the strawberry jelly as "energy-dense," meaning it has a ton of "energy" in the form of calories, but they are the dreaded and incredibly unhealthy and harmful "empty calories" that we often hear about but might not fully understand what is meant by "empty."

When we say "empty calories," all it means is that the calories contain no nutrients (are not nutrient-dense), and when we give our bodies empty calories that have no nutritional value, the only thing our bodies can do with those calories is turn them into fat cells. More fat cells is, for most of us, the exact opposite of what we want for our bodies. So why does the standard American diet (SAD for short, and sad for real) consist mainly of empty calories, with almost no emphasis at all on nutrient density? Because that is what is cheap to produce, easy to market and sell, and makes the most money for large corporations. I'm not going to get too much into the greed/money-making/heartless/inhuman side of why what is promoted as a healthy diet in this world today is what it is, mainly because I'd need a whole other book to get through it all.

What I will say about this sad state of affairs is that about 80% of what is available for purchase in the average American supermarket is not only not whole foods, but is also not nutrient dense. As if that's not bad enough, in most cases, this 80% of what is being sold to us isn't even really food, but instead consists of food-like substances that have been deemed safe for consumption, by people who are, in most cases, completely unqualified in the realm of nutrition and who unfortunately are much more focused on profit than the health of humanity. So what does this mean for us, for the people who want to treat our bodies well, nutritionally, who want to know what is in our food and where it is coming from?

It means that we must be educated and vigilant, and we must read nutrition and ingredient labels. We must stand guard at the door of our mouths, because at the end of the day, we are the ones who get to make the final decisions about what does and does not go in there. No matter how much enticing advertising we see, how many incredible sales there are on crappy food-like products, or how many misleading labels we read (words like "farm fresh" and "all-natural" quite literally mean nothing, and are just used to try to convince consumers that we are buying something that is healthy), we are the gatekeepers, we control the velvet rope and what gets in behind it, and that is an immense amount of power and responsibility that we all have to ourselves, whether we want it or not.

For me, the easiest way to know whether or not a food is nutrient dense is to think about where it came from. Again, using the same example as above, the cup of strawberries grew directly out of the Earth (of course, they were shipped to the supermarket, but especially if they are organic, that is about all they have gone through to get from where they grew to your mouth). But the cup of strawberry jelly went through much more. The strawberries were heavily processed, mashed up, heated, sugar and other ingredients were added, it was jarred, etc. Identifying what the food went through to get to you will almost always be the best and simplest way of knowing if the food is a whole food and whether or not it is nutrient dense.

When we get ourselves to a point where about 80% or more of what we eat consists of nutrient-dense whole foods, our body systems will be well taken care of and have the best ability to operate optimally, and our ability to better manage our blood sugars will be much more consistent. Counting calories won't be as important, because we know that we are choosing nutrients, not empty calories. Getting to this point is part of the journey to improving our health, to being a slightly better version of ourselves each day, each week, each month, each year. Living our own individualized, sustainable healthy lifestyles is not about one single end result. It is about a multitude of amazing benefits that continue to manifest, as long as we stay on the journey.

Nutritional health is a gift that we can choose to give ourselves every single day, an epic journey that we have the privilege to be on if we so choose, a gift we all deserve. And just like any epic journey, there will be bumps in the road, challenges to overcome, villains that will try to foil our efforts, and setbacks that will get in our way and make it seem like we may never get to Mordor—I mean, optimal health. But that is part of any epic journey. Epic journeys offer incredible rewards, new experiences that allow us to learn and grow, introduce us to new friends, and most importantly of all, allow us to see and appreciate ourselves for the incredible warriors we all are. Epic journey------>Epic rewards------>Epic self-love.

Cheat Meals

"Cheat meal" is a term that has gained a lot of popularity in the past 5-10 years, and a practice that has proven to be an incredibly helpful tool to have in our arsenal, if we choose to use it wisely. The only thing that I don't love about it is its name. The word "cheat" implies a negative connotation: cheating on a test, cheating on a significant other. It tells our brains that we are inherently doing something wrong, and that just isn't the case here.

The mindsets we have around food are incredibly important, so I don't like introducing a term like "cheat" into our brain's already very busy schedule of figuring things out. However, I haven't come up with a better name for it yet, so I guess for now, it is what it is. Maybe you can come up with a less negative term for it? If so, tweet me (**@diabetesdomin8r**) your suggestions so I can get the term out of my vocabulary, too! Call it what you want: cheat meal, treat meal, splurge meal, satisfy-your-cravings meal. No matter what name we give it, it means the same thing, and I'm a big fan of using the concept of a cheat meal to our advantage, in a conscious and intentional manner, when creating a sustainable healthy nutritional lifestyle.

What I mean by "cheat meal" might not be the same as others' definitions, but I see it as a moderate splurge that we plan to have once a week in order to satisfy any cravings we might have. The benefits of this are numerous. First, it allows our mindset around food to be more relaxed, if we know that the thing we are craving that isn't nutrient dense or beneficial to our bodies (pizza, doughnuts, chips, ice cream, etc.) isn't off the table for good, and is in fact more than okay to have once a week.

Secondly, and my favorite benefit, is that it helps us to build our WILLPOWER. One of the most common things I hear from people regarding the reason living a healthy nutritional lifestyle hasn't worked for them in the past is because they just don't have strong enough willpower to say "no" to unhealthy foods if they are around them. Willpower is exactly like a muscle; the more consistently we work it, the stronger it becomes, and the less we work it, the weaker it becomes. Most people's willpower muscle is atrophied due to lack of consistent training, but the good news is that anyone can exercise this muscle, no matter their physical fitness level.

There are no injuries that can prevent us from flexing that willpower muscle, no excuses not to make it the strongest muscle we have. As far as the cheat meal concept goes, when we are craving something and are able to tell ourselves that we can have it in a few days, that is a huge exercise for our willpower, and the more often we do it, the stronger our willpower will become. Waiting a mere few days is also something that our brains can get on board with, since it's not like we're saying that we have to wait months to satisfy that craving, just a few days. And if the craving is completely ruling our thoughts to the point that we can't get things done, we have the power to choose to have our cheat meal earlier in the week (but in most cases, our brains would rather wait until the weekend).

Waiting a few days to indulge is doable if the desire to create new habits is real. The other thing that is important to remember when it comes to cheat meals is that it is one meal, not an entire day. That's where the planning ahead and being deliberate and conscious about our decisions really comes into play. It's too easy to let one meal turn into two meals, and two meals into an entire day. Then one day turns into two, and two days turns into a week, and then all of a sudden, things are out of control and we're back in our old patterns. That's why I say a cheat meal is a powerful tool as long as we choose to use it wisely.

Shame around food is something that I dealt with on a very personal level for many years, as I've found it to be for countless people living with diabetes, and I've found that moderation in all things as consistently as possible is the way I was able to work through my issues with feeling that painful shame, embarrassment, and a myriad of other negative feelings around the subject of food. Depending on that cheat meal to completely go insane and gorge is a habit that can too easily become the norm (something I did for a while in the process of implementing cheat meals into my routine, due to my old patterns), and that is something that I want to bring up so that we can be aware of the reality of it.

What I mean by "moderation" is not depriving myself of anything, whether it is cheat meal day or not, but knowing that if I am choosing to eat something that consists mainly of empty calories, I will consciously and proactively portion it out into one serving and move on. I will not give it any more thought cycles, the issue will be closed. The only time this becomes something I really need to put into practice is outside of my own home, like at a birthday or holiday party, or while out to eat with people who might not share my desire to eat healthy.

The reason this isn't an issue in my own home is because I refuse to keep any foods that are unhealthy in my home, for the simple fact that if it is there, I will eat it. This is such an incredibly simple concept that has worked wonders on my ability to sustain my healthy eating lifestyle. If it is within arm's reach, I will eat it. I could still to this day very easily eat myself stupid if I let my guard down and was behind closed doors in my home. I could easily eat an entire package of cookies and more without blinking an eye if it was available to me, and I was sitting in front of the TV and distracted from reality.

That's why it is so imperative that we don't allow these kinds of foods into our homes, where we can so easily slip into mindless, distracted, TV-watching eating mode. Even with all the knowledge and experience I have, and all the work I've put in, I still to this day (and I imagine I will need to for the rest of my life, and I'm okay with that) need to be vigilant when it comes to keeping junky foods out of my own home. I used to binge eat in private every single day for over six years. It became a habit, just like any other, a routine that became a staple in my life. It was a part of my day that I could always depend on and very often look forward to, even though I knew how horrible I would feel afterwards. It was truly a vicious cycle.

I would hide the food from my mom in my bedroom, wait until she was asleep (and/or while she was still at work when I got home from school), and then bring the food out so I could sit in front of the TV and gorge myself on everything from cookies to doughnuts to other carb-filled pastries, candy, or whatever else I decided I wanted to comfort myself that day. Then I would go to sleep full of processed foods, and wake up feeling like total crap, bloated, lacking energy, and with blood sugars through the roof.

Repeating that cycle for so long made it part of my identity, part of who I was. I used to be SO ashamed of that part of my life, so angry for allowing myself to let that continue for so long. It took a long time for me to feel comfortable even saying the words out loud: I binge ate in private. It was my dirty little secret that, for so long, I kept to myself and nobody knew about. It really was both a physical and mental burden.

But when I finally did begin talking about it, I immediately felt relief, even though I was nowhere near being fully recovered from the strong desire to binge whenever anything didn't go my way. **This is why more than anything else, more important than cheat meals or nutrient density or whole foods or anything, I want to say that we MUST recognize and acknowledge if we are caught in a similar pattern that could be defined in any capacity as an eating disorder.**

Please don't suffer in silence for as long as I did. Please don't bear that burden on your own. And please don't expect anyone else to notice and come to save you, especially if you work to keep it hidden. Find somebody who you trust, and talk about it. If you aren't ready to talk about it with someone you know personally, seek counseling through health insurance if that is an option, or check out the website of my dear friend and sister in diabetes and eating disorder recovery, Asha Brown (**http://www.wearediabetes.org**), where you can be connected with the help you need without judgement.

We cannot start creating a sustainable healthy nutritional lifestyle if we are in denial about having a problem as serious as an eating disorder; trust me, I know. What I can tell you is that a full recovery is very possible, and that the learning and growing involved is a beautiful and empowering experience, albeit painful to deal with, especially in the beginning. Now, if I want to have a piece of chocolate and it's not my cheat meal day, I have it (outside of my house) and I don't think twice about it anymore, because I choose to have it in moderation instead of completely binging like I did for so many years.

That took a long time and a lot of practice, but now my relationship with food is something that brings me joy, and something I take immense pride in because I had to fight so hard to achieve it. More than anything, it is crucial to acknowledge our emotional issues around food without blaming or shaming ourselves, and then take it one day at a time, and consistently practice making that willpower muscle stronger and stronger.

One other thing. All of the nutrition information and advice I provide is pertinent for any person who wants to create a sustainable healthy nutritional lifestyle, not just people with diabetes. For some reason, it annoys me when I see foods or recipes labeled "diabetes friendly." The foods that are "friendly" for people with diabetes to eat are the same for those who don't have diabetes. If it's not "diabetes friendly," it's not "friendly" in general! Now let's dive deeper into each of the macronutrients, so we can better understand how to make this nutrient dense whole foods thing work for us!

Carbohydrates: As all of us living with diabetes know, carbohydrates are the macronutrients that have the biggest effect not only on our blood sugar management, but also on our weight management. Each of the three macronutrients have a large variety of sources, some that are very healthy, some that are very unhealthy, and some that are somewhere in between. When it comes to identifying which carbohydrates are the best for our health (meaning the ones that A: have the most nutrients, and B: have the kindest possible impact on our blood sugar levels, it will serve us best in the long run to get a basic understanding of the glycemic index.

To put it super simply (the way I like things to be!), healthy carbs (low glycemic index carbs), when eaten by a human whose pancreas functions normally (aka not a person with diabetes), will cause a slow rise in blood sugar that is easy for the body to process and assimilate by releasing a small amount of insulin. Unhealthy carbs (high glycemic index carbs) cause a much more rapid spike in blood sugar levels, which causes the pancreas to essentially work harder and produce more insulin.

The example I like to use is one that I've tested on myself more than once, because years ago, I was on the fence regarding whether or not the glycemic index really made any difference in blood sugar management and insulin needs. I set up the experiment as accurately as I could, testing the theory at the same time on different days (lunchtime), making sure my blood sugar was in the 90-110 mg/dL range with a straight-ahead facing arrow on my Dexcom. If I eat approximately 30 grams of carbs from a medium-sized pear, I need about 2 units of insulin to cover those carbs. Alternatively, if I eat 30 grams of carbs from Skittles, which ends up being a little less than a ¼-cup serving (keep in mind that the grams of carbs are almost exactly the same; it's the SOURCE of the carbs that is the defining factor here), I need about 3.75 units of insulin to cover that same amount of carbs.

This is due to the glycemic index of each of these items. The GI of a pear is 38 out of 100, while the GI of Skittles is approximately 75 out of 100. At first glance, it might be easy to think that requiring less than two units more of insulin isn't a big deal; however, when we are eating high glycemic index carbs as the majority of our carb intake, those two units end up adding up to many, many more units over the course of a day, week, month, year, and lifetime. Healthy (low GI) carbs require us to take less insulin/medication, and unhealthy carbs (high GI) require us to take more insulin/medication to mitigate the blood sugar spikes, even when the grams of carbs consumed are exactly the same. And as many of us are acutely aware already, insulin and body fat are directly related, especially for people with diabetes. The more insulin we have in our bodies, the more fat our bodies will have the ability to store.

The good news is that it's not important to memorize the GI, we just need to get a handle on the basics.

- The glycemic index (GI) is a scale that goes from 0-100.

- Foods that rank from 1-40 are lower GI foods.

- Foods that rank from 40-60 are middle-range GI foods.

- Foods that rank from 60-100 are high GI foods.

A really easy rule of thumb that covers a ton of categories is that almost all vegetables, fruits, nuts, seeds, beans, and meats are lower on the glycemic index. Are you starting to see a connection here? Most foods that are nutrient-dense, whole foods are lower on the GI. Even the fruits that are a bit higher on the glycemic index (banana, watermelon, mango, pineapple), if eaten in moderation and covered properly by insulin/medication, shouldn't be a problem since they are nutrient-dense, whole foods that contain fiber and water.

Alternatively, processed foods in their traditional forms such as bread, pasta, white rice, bagels, waffles, pancakes, cakes, cookies, muffins, doughnuts, crackers, pretzels, chips and other bagged snacks, juice, and soda all rank higher on the GI. Again, keep in mind that these are all energy-dense foods, full of empty calories, and very low, if not completely devoid of, actual nutrients. I say "in their traditional forms" because there is almost always a delicious, healthy, low GI replacement for just about everything I listed above. Ezekiel brand bread, which can be found in the frozen/health-food section of many stores, still has carbs (and is not gluten-free, in case that is a concern), but it is much healthier than any traditional bread and is low GI, whereas traditional breads are all high GI.

And now that the paleo lifestyle has gained so much popularity, there is an endless resource of recipes online that allow us to recreate just about any tempting treat in a way that is low GI, and in many cases, also gluten- and dairy-free. I'm not saying paleo is the sure way to go, I'm just saying that some recipes labeled as paleo offer healthier versions of certain traditionally prepared dishes. Check out the Recipe section towards the end of this book to see some of my favorite quick, healthy, and low GI recipes!

I'm not about deprivation, and I never promote a nutritional lifestyle that is restrictive, because I strongly believe that being happy and satisfied with what we are eating is key to sustaining a healthy-eating lifestyle. What I do believe in is opening our minds to new experiences (meaning not saying "I don't like that" or "that sounds weird" if we've never tried it), and replacing unhealthy "traditional" versions of certain foods with much healthier, upgraded versions. Replace Triscuits (or other heavily processed crackers) with Mary's Gone Crackers. Replace pasta with spaghetti squash or zucchini noodles. Replace white rice with brown rice or quinoa. Replace grain-based flours (white & wheat) with nut/bean-based flours, like coconut, almond, chickpea, etc. Make your own orange soda with seltzer, the juice of a fresh orange, and a packet of stevia; or make a lemon-lime version by replacing the juice of the orange with the juice of a lemon and a lime.

For more replacement suggestions, go to my website, diabetesdominator.com, and download my Top 50 Healthy and Unhealthy Foods guides (for free) to use a quick reference for what ingredients are the best choices, and which ones to stay away from. When it comes to the glycemic index, nutrient density, and whole foods, I really believe that defaulting to logic and common sense is always our best bet. Once we understand the difference between whole foods and processed foods, we can almost always correctly guess whether it is low or high on the GI.

Just like anything else when it comes to our health, this is not an exact science, just a really helpful guideline that can make all the difference in the world when it comes to seeing blood sugars in the ranges we desire. As a very general rule, most people with diabetes who are not athletes, long-distance runners/bikers, or bodybuilders (I eat about 80-100 grams of carbs per day) do not need more than 100-130 grams of carbohydrates per day. When I say "don't need," I mean do not output enough energy to utilize more than that many carbs in one day.

Any carbs that we consume and don't use for energy are converted into fat cells, meaning we aren't using them for energy. You don't have to be a mad scientist like me; all that is required is paying closer attention to where the foods you eat are coming from. When we pay closer attention, our awareness changes. And once our awareness about anything changes, meaning we simply know a little more about it than we did before, our decisions about that thing will automatically be altered, whether we are conscious of it or not. Changing awareness equals changing decisions.

For example, if you heard a rumor that someone had a bug in their food from a restaurant that you absolutely LOVE, even if you weren't thinking about it on any regular basis, you would most likely choose not to go there, simply because you are aware of the possibility that they might have a bug problem, and you don't want to experience that. Similarly, if you take the exact same route home from work every day, but you heard there was a lot of traffic going that way on your way out of the office, being aware of that would most likely change your decision about which way you take to get home, again, because you don't want to sit in traffic. The same goes for the foods we eat. Once we become more aware of the impact that certain carb sources have on our blood sugars, we will most likely not choose those high-impact foods as often as we used to, because we don't want to deal with the roller-coaster blood sugar fallout.

Before I move on to the next macronutrient, I have a few words about soda, juice, and "sugar-free" or "diet" options of just about anything. Like I said above, I don't like to say "never" because I know from personal experience with myself and through working with so many people over the years that restriction causes psychological fallout, spurring our brains to want these things even more, and that leads us to drive ourselves crazy. As far as juice is concerned, it is never a healthy option unless you are making the juice yourself at home, or are buying freshly-made juice from a juice bar. Any juice that is packaged has been pasteurized, which kills off any of the vitamins and minerals that were in the original fruit that our bodies can actually use. Save the juice for lows, and if it is something you absolutely love, have it once a week for a treat.

The consumption of any sugary, processed drinks on any regular basis will never be a nutritionally-dense choice that will benefit our internal environments. This includes juice, soda, Gatorade and other sports drinks, and the list could go on and on. We are often led to believe that sugar-free versions of traditionally unhealthy foods such as candy, cookies, or soda, for example are healthier for our bodies than the originals, and are a smart way for us to replace those items. Unfortunately, like most things that seem too good to be true, this is the case here as well.

Sugar-free and diet versions of anything are not a healthy replacement for the traditional item, and in some cases, are even more damaging to our internal environments than the regular version, due to the laundry list of processed chemicals, additives, and preservatives. Aspartame is one of the most heavily researched food additives by both the FDA and thousands of other independent labs in history, due to continuing controversy over a myriad of horrible health problems that may be caused or exacerbated by consistent consumption of aspartame, including cancer and multiple sclerosis.

For the most part, as many people with diabetes know, unless we are elite athletes, eating a diet that consists of 45-60 grams of carbs per meal plus multiple snacks that consist of 25 grams of carbs each isn't a healthy diet. However, check out the following website for the nutritional guidelines set forth by the American Diabetes Association, the most trusted source for diabetes information nationwide, who are still recommending that high level of carbohydrate intake for people with diabetes, even now that we know so much more about how carbs affect our blood sugar levels: **http://www.diabetes.org/mfa-recipes/about-our-meal-plans.html**

What does this have to do with aspartame? My point with this comparison is to be aware that the information given to us by large companies, corporations, or federal government agencies is not always correct or healthy, and in some cases, can be outright dangerous and detrimental to our health. I can say with certainty that aspartame breaks down into methyl alcohol (wood alcohol), which converts to formaldehyde in the human body, and I don't know about you, but the thought of ingesting formaldehyde on any consistent basis is a scary and disturbing thought.

I'm not going to go much deeper into this, as it is a lengthy and controversial topic, but I will say that after eight plus years of doing my own research, I fully believe that aspartame is poison and poses a real threat of throwing off our internal chemistry and building up in our cells over time, which creates a weakened internal environment that is ideal for any number of other health problems to manifest. Again, just like everything else, this is a choice we all must make for ourselves. The following is a link to more information regarding the dangers of aspartame:
http://articles.mercola.com/sites/articles/archive/2012/11/11/aspartame-dangers.aspx

I recommend treating sugar-free and diet versions of any item the same way you would treat the real thing: only have it on rare occasions. Those of us living with chronic diseases already have enough pressure on our internal environments to try to stay balanced without throwing a slew of harmful additives into the mix and hoping our bodies can figure out how to process them. The bottom line is that sugar-free and diet versions are not healthier, or safer choices. So what are we supposed to eat then?

Every day, there are more and more companies and products coming into the marketplace that are fully health-conscious and know that we are out here wanting TRULY healthier versions of some of our favorite treats without added chemicals, additives, and preservatives. Some of my favorites are PUR Gum, Zevia soda, and Lily's chocolate bars. When it comes to chocolate, I'm a big fan of organic dark chocolate (the darker the better, 85% or so) as a great way to satisfy sweet cravings without adding many carbs to the mix, and also getting the benefit of fiber. There are a number of great options to use as sugar substitutes, ones that are derived from plants. My favorite (and most widely available and recognizable) is stevia, and there are also erythritol and xylitol, all available on *Amazon* and other online retailers.

Protein: Just like there are many sources from which carbs can come, the same goes for protein. And just like carbs, some sources of protein are much healthier for our bodies than others. There are a variety of stances in the health and fitness world on how much protein a human being needs each day. In my opinion, just like everything else nutrition-related, protein needs will vary from person-to-person, depending on genetics, internal chemistry, individual goals, activity level/type/duration, and just plain old personal preferences.

I work out six days a week, which usually consists of a mix of heavy and fast-paced weight lifting/resistance training, or low-rep heavy weight lifting, yoga, and cardio in some form, such as walking, jogging, intervals, or Zumba. On average, I eat anywhere from 60-90 grams of protein per day, trying to focus on being closer to the upper range on the days I lift weights, but I don't always make it. This is what works for me, and I've tried many different protocols over the years. Some experts say that we need one gram of protein per pound of bodyweight, and other experts say women need a minimum of 46 grams of protein per day, and men need a minimum of 56 grams of protein per day.

Obviously, even experts have wildly differing opinions on what is ideal. There is no expert that is more qualified to decide how much protein you need each day than YOU. This is a personal decision that should be made after experimenting while keeping a food journal (much more on how to keep an easy food journal coming up), and seeing how you feel with different levels of protein intake.

I have eaten meat in some form or another almost my whole life (with a few stints eating a vegetarian and, at times vegan, diet). However, as I get older and healthier, I find that the less often I eat meat, the more energy I have, the clearer my mind is, and the better I feel overall. When I do eat meat, it is only from grass-fed or organic sources. I choose to eat only organic, or pastured eggs. I choose to eat only wild-caught fish—no farm-raised fish until there are much tighter rules and regulations on how farm-raised fisheries are operated and monitored regarding over-crowding and antibiotic use.

When choosing to eat meat, the most important thing to do is consider the source. When we ingest meat that has been treated with hormones, antibiotics, contains nitrates, nitrites, or anything else that pollutes the animal's internal environment, it also pollutes our internal environments.

The most common opposition to choosing organic, grass-fed meats is that it's too expensive. I agree that it is more expensive than its polluted counterparts; however, I believe that when we choose to put our health and the health of our loved ones at the top of our list of priorities, this is a necessary step to take, and one that requires us to take a step back, take a much closer look at and examine our budgets in order to make work. The best and easiest solution is to eat meat less often, and when we do eat it, eat less of it.

Explore meal options where meat is not the centerpiece but a sidebar, or even non-existent (things like chili or soups where you can easily use much less meat, or none at all). At the end of the day, health is the foundation for all happiness, and without feeling healthy on a consistent basis, it is difficult to lead a happy, fulfilling existence. And it can be difficult to create a healthy internal environment when polluted sources of meat are being introduced on a consistent basis.

When we begin to make healthy, sustainable changes, we often begin to understand that even if we have to cut back erroneous spending a bit or eat meat less often, the nourishment that goes into our bodies is non-negotiable and does not come second to anything (other than medications that keep us alive), because food is medicine. All too often, we think that choosing organic, grass-fed, non-GMO food options are too expensive in the moment, but I see it as a case of either paying for it now with money, or paying for it later with any number of serious health problems.

And let's face it, no matter our income, just about every one of us spends money on things that don't benefit our health, like smoking, drinking, too many pairs of shoes, or Starbucks every day. I believe that if we challenge ourselves to lay out a monthly budget plan, we will very often find an area (or two) where we can cut back, organize better, or prioritize differently in order to provide our bodies with the level of nutrition it deserves as often as possible. I'm not saying that it is the end of the world if we eat non-organic or non-grass-fed meat on occasion–I do it too–but the goal is to keep it to a minimum and choose the healthy options when it is in our control to do so as often as possible.

We truly are what we eat. The quality of food that we choose to put into our bodies will ultimately determine our quality of health, and will also be reflected in the way we look on the outside. Food is the best and safest form of medicine, if we take the time to learn how to use it to our advantage. For me, this goes even further than the fact that I know how intensely polluted the non-organic, non-grass-fed meats are.

I am a crazy animal person in general. At times, I love animals more than I love people…I know I'm not alone on this! The animals that are not raised on organic/grass-fed farms are treated so horribly that it actually makes me sick to my stomach, and I cry if I think about it too much. I've watched so many documentaries on the subject, because I am so passionate about knowing where my food comes from (please watch *Food, Inc.* to get more educated on the reality of factory farms, as well as *Forks Over Knives, Cowspiracy, and Earthlings*), and have seen with my own eyes the horror-shows that are factory farms.

Cows with giant holes cut into their sides so that more food than they can eat with their mouths can be pumped into their stomachs through a tube so they get bigger faster. Chickens that are packed together so tightly that they are literally standing on top of each other in their own waste. Chickens routinely have their beaks violently snapped off so that food literally can be poured into their mouths faster than they can eat it naturally, again, so that they can make them bigger faster. Animals being beaten until bloody, just to get them to move from one place to another because they are so sick and abused they can barely move.

These things are routine practices, not just something that happens now and then. These are the things of twisted horror movies. Things we don't like to think or talk about because they are so incredibly disturbing on so many levels. Creating a sustainable healthy, nutritional lifestyle sometimes requires us to get real and allow ourselves to be exposed to realities about which we might not want to hear. These realities are some of the many factors involved in why I don't eat meat every day, and when I do, I make it a very high priority to choose meat that comes from more humane sources, no matter what the cost.

134

There are a wide variety of great sources of protein that don't come from animals. I eat nuts and seeds and/or almond or peanut butter every day. One really important factor to pay attention to when buying nut or seed butters is to check the ingredient label, especially when it comes to peanut butter. Choose organic when possible, but even more importantly, make sure there is only one ingredient on the label, either almonds or peanuts (and salt if you like it a little saltier).

Mostly all of the more popular brands of peanut butter like Jif, Skippy, and Smuckers, etc., all have a bunch of unnecessary and unhealthy ingredients added into their peanut butter, like palm oil and high fructose corn syrup. A couple of brands I use are Nature's Promise and Crazy Richard's. All beans, such as black beans, white beans, lima beans, lentils, chickpeas (hummus), peas, sun-dried tomatoes, leafy greens; all raw nuts/seeds and nut/seed butters; and quinoa are just some examples of excellent sources of protein.

I also supplement my protein with vegetarian protein powder. Right now, my favorites that I think taste the best are Vega One, Vega Sport, and MRM Veggie Elite. I have tried some of the raw vegetarian protein such as Sun Warrior, and although I think it is an excellent product, I couldn't get over the way it tasted. So, I go with what I like and you should do the same. A quick note on soy-based products like tofu and tempeh: just like anything else, we must consider the source. I only choose soy products on occasion, and only ones that are organic and non-GMO.

At the end of the day, it is best to choose as many organic products as possible, including fruits and vegetables, as they are exposed to so many pesticides and toxins. However, even if we eat all of these things and they aren't organic/grass-fed/non-GMO, we will still be MUCH better off and much healthier in general. Eating a diet that consists mainly of the non-organic/non-grass-fed/non-GMO version of any fruit or vegetable or meat is still much healthier than eating a diet that consists mainly of processed, non-nutrient-dense foods, such as fast foods, frozen dinners, canned meals/soups, packaged noodles, or really anything so heavily processed that it can sit stored on a shelf for extended periods of time. It really comes down to choosing to do what works best for you right now, and being willing to make small changes over the course of time. But first and foremost, always choose to eat whole, real, nutrient-dense foods in their natural (unprocessed) states the majority of the time.

Fat: On any given day, my diet consists of 50-60% fat. Sometimes when I say this, people look incredulous, like they can't believe I'm fit and healthy and eat so much fat every day. Fat has been put through the wringer as far as being blamed for the world's obesity epidemic and other weight-related health issues, when in reality, especially for people with diabetes, excess processed carbohydrates and sugar are really to blame. The truth is that healthy fats are just that–healthy–and super beneficial to our bodies.

Selecting foods that are rich in monounsaturated and polyunsaturated fats, and saturated fats from plant sources versus trans fats puts us on track to being a fat-burning machine. The human body must ingest fat to burn fat. When we're not taking in enough fat, our bodies will instinctually hold on to the fat it has, due to the fact that it's not getting enough healthy fat consistently, and it doesn't want to let go of its precious reserves. When we start consistently giving our bodies the healthy fats they need, they will more willingly let go of reserved fat because they are confident more will be coming their way soon. The healthiest fats generally come from plant sources, although there are some animal sources that offer health benefits as well.

Healthy fats include: avocados; coconut flesh; unsweetened full-fat coconut milk (Native Forest is the brand I use); raw nuts and seeds; single-ingredient nut/seed butters; plant-based, cold-pressed oils such as extra virgin olive oil, avocado oil, almond oil, walnut oil, sesame oil, pumpkin seed oil, and coconut oil, to name a few. Animal sources of healthy fat include wild-caught fatty fish such as salmon, tuna, and sardines, as well as organic/pastured egg yolks, grass-fed/organic meats (lean cuts), and organic ghee.

You may have noticed that I didn't include cheese or dairy here in any capacity. Although I do fully understand the desire to eat cheese regularly (I love cheese; it's delicious and it's low carb, so I totally get it), over the years, I have weaned myself off of eating it on a regular basis. Instead, I save it for a cheat meal or treat it the same way I would treat any other highly processed food, and only eat it occasionally, being very conscious to portion out and eat only one serving (moderation), because I know it is highly processed and super salty, and thus does not offer healthy fat.

If you are a cheese-aholic like I used to be, and you want to try to start eating it less often, take it slowly. Have a sprinkle of cheese on a salad instead of sitting down and eating a whole block at once (something I've done many times). And when we eat a smaller amount at a time, it will be easier to buy a local, organic cheese instead of a bag of shredded, processed cheese. Maybe make it a longer-term goal to work on for the future (or not); it really is a matter of finding the nutritional lifestyle that works best for you and is sustainable.

When it comes to milk, it isn't something that I choose to include in my diet at all, for a number of reasons. Dairy is not a food group, it is not a substance that the human body needs to thrive in any way. If nobody in the world ever ate dairy (from farm animals) again, nobody would suffer any adverse health issues due to its absence. Milk is a high glycemic index carb, and it is also very heavily processed to get from the cow to our glass.

I take pride in being as logical as possible and depending on common sense to help me figure things out when I'm not 100% sure, or if I think the information I'm being given might be wrong, so here is my logical thought process regarding milk. Milk is designed by God or nature or Gaia or whatever you believe, in order to allow the cows' calves (baby cows) to grow approximately two pounds per day, 730 pounds per year, until they are no longer drinking cow's milk. Why in the world would we, as humans, drink the breast milk of another creature that was designed to make the drinker of that milk gain weight at that pace?

It just doesn't make any sense to me whatsoever. Additionally, about 75% of the world's population is genetically unable to properly digest milk and other dairy products. We label this as a diagnosable condition called "lactose intolerance," when in reality, *most* humans lack the enzymes needed to properly digest milk. Humans require the lactase enzyme to digest milk, and in most humans, this enzyme dies off as toddlers grow into adolescents.

Most of us living with diabetes try to limit weight gain, and also try to limit our intake of high glycemic carbs. This is another case, like any other, where each of us must make our own decisions. I, however, implore you to defer to your common sense on this one.

This is another example of how the information coming from large corporations or government agencies might not be correct or the healthiest information.

Unhealthy fats include: non-grass-fed/non-organic animal meat (especially fattier cuts); cheese; anything deep-fried; processed oils such as canola, vegetable, corn, Crisco; non-grass-fed butter; margarines like I Can't Believe It's Not Butter; heavily salted and/or roasted-with-added-oil nuts and seeds (look for the term "dry-roasted," or read the ingredient label to see if any other oils are listed); nut or seed butters that have ingredients on the label other than the nut or seed from which it is made and salt, candy, cookies, cakes, pastries, and ice cream. Again, just because they aren't necessarily healthy doesn't mean that they aren't fine to have in moderation now and then, just like any other processed, empty calorie foods.

The movement towards eating healthier, more locally-sourced, sustainable ingredients is growing every day, and food manufacturers are listening to the demands of their customers. With ingredients like coconut oil, coconut milk, coconut/almond flour, unsweetened cocoa powder, Frontier vanilla extract, stevia, and avocados, we have the ability to make an endless number of incredibly delicious recipes that are actually good for us!

Just use our friend *Google* to search for recipes for paleo desserts, for example, which will give us the ability to recreate just about any sweet treat that we love in a much healthier way. Just remember to go light on any maple syrup or honey that the recipes might suggest; try halving it and adding stevia to compensate. Don't be afraid to get in the kitchen and experiment! Learning how to create healthy meals and desserts is one of the most fun, empowering, and creative aspects of growing into our own sustainable healthy lifestyles.

Keeping a Food Journal: You Can't Manage What You Don't Measure

Please visit <u>diabetesdominator.com/bookresources</u> to view screenshots of my MFP food journal.

In order to set a baseline, to have a real idea and visual representation of how much we are eating and where the calories are coming from, and to make intelligent decisions about what the best next steps are for our nutritional lifestyle, we must keep a daily food journal. This is where the rubber meets the road and things get real. Having a visual representation of what we consume is so helpful for a number of reasons.

First, when we can actually see what the foods (and drinks) we are consuming contain as far as calories, carbs, protein, fat, sodium, and fiber (which are the categories that I think are the most important to pay attention to), our awareness automatically begins to change. We begin to learn more than we knew before, whether we are trying to or not, because we are seeing it before our very eyes. The only way we won't get a fairly accurate representation of what we eat is if we choose to omit things because seeing it staring us in the face can be painful and we'd rather forget that we ate them (been there, done that!)

Keeping a food journal, at least until we feel confident in our nutritional decisions and get into a groove, is crucial. And even when we feel like we have the hang of things it's important not to get too overconfident too quickly and lose sight of the foundations we build our nutritional habits off of. We can't find the way to where we want to go if we don't look at where we are now and correct our course accordingly. Eventually, we have to come out of autopilot, and keeping a food journal is the most beneficial place to start.

This is where www.myfitnesspal.com (which I refer to as MFP) comes into play. In my opinion, MFP is by far, no contest, the most valuable free health management tool available on the internet today. The site makes it simple to keep track of everything we eat, with an incredibly extensive database of foods. There is even a barcode scanner built into the cellphone application, and as long as what we are eating has a barcode (even bags of spinach, apples, or other healthy foods have barcodes these days), we can scan it right in and adjust for the portion we ate in a matter of seconds.

When we choose to familiarize ourselves with and use MFP daily (and honestly) until we have adopted our own sustainable healthy nutrition habits and feel fully confident and empowered with our nutritional decisions, we are choosing to win. Eventually, it won't be as imperative to use it every day, because our nutrition choices will become more habitual. But it is still always good to check-in to make sure we are where we want to be, and so that we know our bodies are receiving the nutrients they need to help us thrive.

One very important thing to keep in mind is that not all entries in MFP are 100% accurate, because they are entered by random people around the world, and that's okay. Just like all other areas of our lives, we are not going for perfection here. It is much more beneficial to be able to look back and see what we ate, even if the macronutrients in MFP aren't 100% accurate, than to have nothing at all to look at.

When setting up a MFP account, it is imperative that we set our own individualized caloric and macronutrient values based on our own specific needs and goals, versus depending on the computerized guess of what we need, which MFP will automatically provide for us upon setting up an account. A computer's generalized calculations can be an unhealthy plan to follow, especially since MFP often recommends too few calories and WAY too many carbs. I have been using MFP both for myself and with clients for over six years now, so I have become an expert on using the site to our advantage. Luckily, it's not hard to do when you know where to go, so I'm going to give you the insider information on how you can set your own values from the get go, and change them according to how you are feeling and progressing at any time.

This is a step-by-step process, so bear with me as I get into some bullet points here. You must set your values from a regular computer or a laptop, not from a mobile phone. Entering our food from a mobile phone is great, but we can't see the readout of where we are as far as our macronutrients are concerned from the mobile app, so it is important to check-in on a regular computer/laptop each day to get that visual representation of where we are. Here we go!

Reminder: As I stated in the beginning, I am not a medical doctor. Always check with your physician before making any changes to your health and nutrition habits. What I recommend is based on consistently proven, evidence-based results that I have achieved with both myself and hundreds of clients with all types of diabetes.

Just as everything else in the life of a Diabetes Dominator needs regular maintenance and adjustments, our MFP values will likely have to be adjusted/played around with now and then in order to find the most ideal fit for each of our individual lifestyles. Don't be afraid to make changes if you're not seeing the differences you are looking for in your blood sugars after a month or so of consistency. Just like we must be confident in adjusting our own insulin levels based on different day-to-day activities and events that take place in our lives, we must adjust our nutrition accordingly as well. These values will need adjusting if we begin a different or more intense workout routine than we are currently doing, as we need more calories to sustain harder workouts. Our insulin/medication levels will also need adjusting, since once we begin eating mostly nutritionally-dense foods and working out regularly, our insulin/medication needs will change.

First things first, go **to www.myfitnesspal.com** and create an account. Once you have your account, it's time to customize!

- Click "Settings" at the top of the page, then click "Diary Settings."
- Change the "Nutrients Tracked" from the drop-down menus to reflect "Carbohydrates," "Protein," "Fat," "Sodium," and "Fiber," then scroll down to the bottom of the page and click "Save Changes."
- Click "Goals" at the top of the page, then click "Edit" in the "Daily Nutrition Goals" box
- Here is where we customize. First, set your daily calorie goal. A good jumping-off point for most average adult women is 1300-1500 calories, and 1800-2000 calories for most average adult men. I can't stress enough that these are LOOSE guidelines. If you are an athlete, you will need more calories to sustain your activities. If you are mostly sedentary, you may need to err on the lower side.
- Now we set our macronutrient ratios from the drop-down menus. I like to start at about 25-30% carbs, 45-50% fat, and 20-25% protein. Again, this is not concrete and will not be perfect for everyone. These are just suggestions for a place to begin. Once you have the ratios set, scroll down and click "Save Changes" at the bottom of the page.
- Click "Edit" in the "Micronutrients" box.

- Change "Sodium" to 1500-1800 mg, and change "Fiber" to somewhere between 30-40 grams. Scroll down and click "Save Changes" at the bottom of the page.

Now when you click on the "FOOD" tab at the top of the page, you will see your daily goals all lined up in a row at the bottom. I like to think of it as a gamification of our nutritional needs, a kind of plug-and-play to see how we can get the foods we eat to get in the range of the goals we set, and have fun with it in the meantime. I can't stress enough that it's okay if we don't get to the exact values, and it is likely that we will rarely, if ever, hit the mark to a T.

Like I said before, it's not about being perfect, it's about learning and becoming aware of what we are putting into our bodies. Please do not beat yourself up if you don't hit the mark! This tool is meant to be helpful and reduce our stress around food by allowing us to feel confident in what we are putting into our bodies, not to add stress because we are not hitting the mark exactly. And remember that some MFP entries are not 100% accurate, so trying to be perfect with information that isn't accurate is, again, like trying to capture a unicorn; it won't happen, and we will drive ourselves crazy if we keep chasing after something that doesn't exist.

I recommend choosing another app or avenue for tracking exercise, and not entering exercise into MFP because MFP will automatically add additional calories and macronutrients to your daily goals to compensate for the exercise you did, and that's not what we want, particularly if we are looking to lose some body fat. If you are an athlete and not looking to lose body fat, and want to replenish those calories and macros, then by all means, enter your exercise into MFP.

Each person's needs will vary. However, in my experience, an adult female who exercises 3-5 times a week at a moderate intensity (fast walking, light jogging, occasional weight lifting) with any type of diabetes generally does well in the range of 80-120 grams of carbohydrates per day. An adult male who exercises 3-5 times a week at a moderate intensity with any type of diabetes generally does well in the range of 100-140 grams of carbohydrates per day, especially if fat loss and insulin/medication reduction are on the list of goals.

Many things will affect how many calories each person will need day-to-day and in what ratio the macronutrients should be to fill up those calories, including age, goals, frequency and intensity of exercise, intensity of his/her job (sedentary versus manual labor), etc. There is not and will never be a one-size-fits-all number. One thing to be very aware of that I see happen often is going from overeating to undereating once we get into tracking our daily intakes. Undereating is just as detrimental to our bodies as overeating. I'm not sure where the 1200 calorie diet for weight loss standard came from, but 1200 calories is simply not enough, especially if we are exercising, and undereating can very quickly stall any fat loss and put us on the plateau level.

Now that we have the basics of nutrition, we can choose our foods with more confidence, knowing that we have the power to decide where our nutrition comes from and how to make the healthiest choices possible. Keep this up for a few weeks and before you know it, eating healthy will be one of the most beneficial and empowering habits you ever develop.

14

EXERCISE

"Those who think they have no time for exercise will sooner or later have to find time for illness."
-Edward Stanley

As it stands, each of us has only one vehicle to get us through our lives, and that is our physical body. I say "as it stands" because breakthroughs in medical science continue to happen every day. We are now 3-D printing fully functional limbs, and people get major organ transplants every day (my sister had a liver transplant five years before she passed away, and one of my clients had a heart transplant and exercises regularly), so maybe someday we will easily be able to swap out our old, rusty parts for shiny new ones (I'm looking forward to the bionic pancreas!) But, until that time comes, we are best served to treat what we have with love and care, especially for those of us living with diabetes.

The incredibly beneficial effects that exercise has on our blood sugar management are kind of profound, if you take a second to think about it. Check out **www.bigbluetest.org** to see what just 14-20 minutes of exercising can do for our blood sugars, pretty much immediately. By entering a few data points (what your blood sugar was before exercising, and what is was after), not only are you contributing to valuable research and doing wonders for your own health, but you are also donating $1 to charities that provide diabetes supplies to those in need. It doesn't get any easier or more beneficial than that! That's one of the best things about exercise—we don't have to wait to see the benefits, they begin to happen right away, and we don't have to do a large amount of it to reap those amazing benefits.

We are all too familiar with the fact that our bodies don't always do what they are supposed to, and that our bodies are both extremely fragile, and incredibly resilient at the same time. Our body is our temple, and the thing on which we depend to allow us to do everything we love and cherish, like playing with our kids, hugging our loved ones, providing for our families, following our passions and dreams, playing with our precious pets.

All too often, we take these amazing, miraculous machines we call bodies for granted, just assuming that they will be there for us to do what we need them to do, when we need them to do it. But the way we treat our bodies as far as physical movement is a two-way street. The human body was designed to move, and move a lot. But if we don't move regularly with intention, our bodies will react in turn.

The less we move, the less our bodies will be capable of allowing us to do. Our bones, joints, tendons, ligaments, and muscles need to be moved on a regular basis so that we can keep depending on them to serve us throughout our lives. The truth is, at some point or another, we all end up treating our bodies poorly in some way.

Many of us fill our bodies full of processed foods as we sit still in front of a computer all day at work, then we come home and do the same thing while sitting on a couch all night, leaving our bodies craving the physical movement that we as humans were designed to perform every single day. Many of us will religiously take our cars to get the oil changed every 3,000 miles, or if something lights up on the dashboard, we immediately make an appointment to get it checked out. But when our one and only body cries out for help, whether through frequent mood swings, feeling lethargic all the time, brain fog, sleeplessness, or achy, stiff joints, we all too often choose to ignore the warning signs for as long as possible, just hoping they will go away. This happens all the time and is disturbing on many levels; cars are replaceable, bodies are not.

Why would we ignore the signs our bodies are always sending out to us? One of the reasons is because we often perceive everything else that is going on around us (our spouses, kids, jobs, caring for others) as more important than caring for our own health. When someone says, "I don't have time to exercise," what they are really saying is that they don't value exercise as a high enough priority to SCHEDULE it into their daily calendar and treat it the same way they would treat a meeting with their boss, which they would be sure not to miss because they know how important it is and that there will be lasting consequences if missed.

For some people (this used to be me), watching TV is much more important than 30 minutes of physical movement. If this is where you are now, you are not alone, and I used to have the exact same mindset. In order to slowly begin to change this mindset and priority structure, we have to take some steps and leaps outside our comfort zones. We have to work on our beliefs one day at a time, until it is part of what we know to be certain that physical movement is more important than TV, video games, emails, social media, or anything else that isn't moving us towards a healthier existence.

We have to commit to making the time to making it happen, and the only way this will come true is if we schedule it into our calendars and PLAN AHEAD. This might not be comfortable, but nothing life-changing ever happens inside our limited comfort zone bubbles. It is only when we step out of that bubble and drop the excuses that real change begins to happen.

And like I said above, the exercise doesn't have to be excessive, incredibly strenuous, or take a huge chunk of time out of the day. I'm not talking about training like an Olympic athlete here; I'm talking about 15-60 minutes of movement, 3-6 times a week. Getting up and doing just ten minutes of movement a few times a day will not only give us those great benefits, but will also help to create the habit more quickly, especially in the beginning, when exercise isn't part of our routine, because the more often we do something, the more our minds will come to expect us to do it again.

It's not as much about duration as it is about frequency, and the truth of the matter is that any movement is always better than none at all. We don't have to have sweat pouring off of us and be unable to breathe to benefit from exercise! Taking a leisurely stroll around the neighborhood, doing 30 minutes of yoga, or doing a few bodyweight exercises in our own homes is all it takes to get into a really great groove and routine, no gym membership required. Building this habit can happen in the time it takes to watch one episode of your favorite show—heck, even doing small bursts of movement during commercials is incredibly beneficial! This is an amount of time we all have somewhere in our lives, whether we are willing to admit it or not, and sometimes admitting that we are not too busy is the hardest obstacle to overcome.

The best thing to do at the beginning is to keep it simple. Don't expect to run a half-marathon or even a 5k if you've never run a day in your life. Aim for a quarter mile, then a half mile, then a mile, then two, then three, and so on, incrementally improving over time, aiming to be just a little stronger than you were the day/week/month before. It's not a bad thing to strive for a big goal, but when we do that in the very beginning, it can be a vicious form of self-sabotage because it is a goal that we can't reach in a timeframe that will satisfy our minds, and that can very easily lead to giving up.

Try a class that you have been thinking about to see if you like it. Even if you don't like it, at least you know now, and got a workout in in the meantime. Or if you like to be outside, commit to taking a walk, or walking with a little jogging interspersed here and there. Or try swimming or bike riding or Zumba. Make it fun, and don't stress about whether or not it's the "right thing" or if it's "enough!" If you're enjoying it, it's enough and it's right!

One other thing that can be a real issue for many of us (and used to be for me) is comparing our results to someone else's. This is a detrimental habit to form, and one that is truly illogical and nonsensical. Nobody else's body is going to progress at the same rate as ours, even if we are doing the exact same workout routine. It's one thing (a great thing) to have a workout buddy or accountability partner; however, it's another thing if we get caught up in comparing our results to theirs and feeling bad about our own efforts that should be celebrated no matter what. As we get further into the six pillars of total health, you will probably notice that they are all very closely intertwined—there is a ton of mindset involved with exercise!

For me, exercise used to be a foreign concept. It was something that I accepted was for other people, but not for me, because I wasn't athletic in my own mind. It was something that I literally never did my entire life until I was 19 years old (which is when I began to dabble), and when I thought about exercise, I would dismiss it just as quickly as it entered my mind because the thought of doing it was embarrassing! I had so many unanswered questions about it: what should I do? Where should I start? How much, and how often? Would I look stupid trying to exercise when I had no clue what I was doing? This was before I stopped worrying about what other people thought about me, specifically when I was doing something that was aimed at improving my health or helping others, but that's another story for another book!

My aversion to exercise started when I was in 6th grade. That's when I started gaining a lot of weight, and I was also much taller than most of the boys and girls in my grade. In gym class, we had to run around the track, among other things, and that was a mortifying experience for me. Things were flopping around (I didn't really have a sports bra at that point), and kids were mean. I was teased relentlessly about my over-developed body and for being overweight.

One kid who shall remain nameless (and trust me, I remember his name, and actually see him on Facebook to this day; that kind of thing really scars a child!) called me "The Fridge" in front of the entire class on a regular basis, which was the nickname for a gigantic football player who played for our home team in Philadelphia growing up. It hurt like hell, was so embarrassing, and made me insanely angry, both at the kids for being so cruel, and at myself for being so much bigger than everyone else. Why was I so different, I wondered? I wanted to crawl into a hole and just be alone.

Kids didn't understand my diabetes, so the fact that I had to eat snacks when they weren't eating, and sometimes drink juice and leave the classroom to eat food only fueled their insults about why I was overweight. This was in the age before the internet. I didn't have access to the internet until I was 15 or 16, and even then, it was just super slow dial-up and the diabetes online community was barely in its infancy at that point, besides the fact that I didn't even think to look for others online who had diabetes. In fact, I didn't ever meet another person who had diabetes until I was in my 20s.

This was before we had a system in place ("Safe at School," through the American Diabetes Association) that provided guidelines regarding kids with diabetes and their rights while in school, which I'm so happy and relieved to see is now a valuable resource for kids and parents today. When I first started exploring exercise as something that I could realistically fit into my life, something inside me began to shift. First, it was just taking walks, which got longer and faster as I became more confident. But then something else happened...I met a boy.

He really helped me get past some of my exercise demons by supporting and encouraging me to put on rollerblades. He was an avid roller hockey player, and about six months after we met, he bought me a pair of rollerblades for Christmas. At first I laughed, really thinking it was some kind of joke, having flashbacks to my grade school exercise-related terrors. But then I realized that he just wanted to invite me more into his world and his love for hockey, and

I decided that even though I had zero confidence in my balance and/or ability to skate, I would allow him to try to teach me, and I would be a good sport about it because he really did care about my health and wellbeing.

You see, we tend to do much more for people we care about than we will ever consider doing for ourselves, so having outside motivation to get moving can be helpful at first. If you don't want to do it for yourself at first, do it for your kids so you can set a good example and they can pick up your healthy habits. Do it for your significant other so you can be the best version of yourself that you can possibly be for them, do it for someone in your family or circle of friends who might not be able to exercise themselves due to any number of reasons.

Then as time goes on and the habit begins to develop, you will want to do it for yourself as well—that's just the way it goes! The first time I put on those skates, it was terrifying, and I felt like a baby animal that was just born and learning to use its legs for the first time. But after time and practice, and after putting a hockey stick in my hands, which made me feel more balanced (and kind of bad-ass!), I started to learn how to rollerblade.

Yes, I fell. And yes, it hurt. And to this day, I don't know how to stop properly without running into a wall! But that didn't matter, because I was having FUN! After a while, I didn't even need him to be with me anymore, I just went out by myself! What a concept. It really was the catalyst for building my confidence about what was possible for me when it came to exercising. Even though the relationship didn't last, and I have no idea where this person is today, I am forever grateful that he gave me that gift. It truly is a gift that keeps on giving, as I am able to help other people begin to embrace their own love of exercise every day.

Fast-forward from age 19, when the exercise spark was lit, to my mid-20s, when I decided to enroll in personal training school. Granted, I was more comfortable with exercise than I was when I first started, but I still couldn't do a single push-up and had only ventured into lifting weights a year or so beforehand thanks to my husband's encouragement and assistance. The reason I enrolled in this completely immersive, 500-hour program was because I was making a living as a personal chef, cooking healthy meals for clients who had a variety of medical issues. Once my clients began eating healthier, they would inevitably ask me what they should do for exercise. At this point, I was a nutritionist and knew my way around how to create a healthy nutritional lifestyle, but I was in no way qualified to be dishing out exercise advice, as I had only been at it for a few years myself and had no real expertise on the subject. So I decided to go get that expertise, and in that six-month process, my life changed again.

My ideas of what was possible changed again as well. I went in scared out of my mind, thinking I would be the only person in the program who wasn't muscle-bound and super well versed in the ways of exercise physiology. But thankfully, I was wrong. Although there were some very experienced people in my class, the majority of us were all after the same thing: to get better at something about which we were growing more and more passionate in our lives.

I went in unable to do a single push up, and came out six months later able to do three sets of ten. Thinking about it still amazes me because the changes happened so much quicker than I ever thought possible, and that was because I practiced consistently, as doing a push-up was one of my top goals. After we learned (in Latin!) every muscle, bone, and joint in the body, and every action they performed, we went right out of the classroom and into the gym to put what we just learned into practice.

We trained our classmates and put them on three-month programs. It was one of the most life-altering six-month periods of my life, and I am forever grateful to my husband for finding this program for me; and moreover, encouraging me to sign up and follow my growing passion for physical fitness. I am also forever grateful to the teacher of that program, Barry Fritz, for being an incredible inspiration, and generous wealth of knowledge and encouragement. His humble attitude and willingness to support all of his students no matter what level they were on still to this day inspires me to model my teaching methods after his examples. The fact that he had a great sense of humor didn't hurt either.

After that six months, I was finally fully confident in my abilities to both tackle any exercise challenge I decided to take on in life, and to help other people find an exercise routine that worked for them and teach them how to do it. I finally embraced that I was not only mentally stronger than I believed I was, but also physically stronger than I ever believed I could be.

Before getting started on any new exercise program, it is crucial to get a notebook, or make a Google Drive spreadsheet specifically for tracking your progress. Again, you can't manage what you don't measure. You will never know how far you have come if you don't know where you started, so consistent tracking is a must for keeping yourself inspired and motivated.

Get a measuring tape and take all of your measurements (including arms, chest, waist, hips, and thighs) and write them down in your notebook or Google Drive document, along with the date and your weight. I recommend taking your measurements once a month to gauge progress; and remember, always measure in the exact same spot on your body each time!

Keeping track of measurements, and also taking photos each month, time-lapse style, is so important because when we start working out, sometimes the number on the scale stays exactly the same for a while because we are both losing fat and gaining muscle at the same time, but our measurements change. We lose inches, we feel more energetic, we sleep better, and our clothes fit better or even get too big, which are the best indicators of the progress we are making.

Another thing that is super helpful in gauging progress is to have a baseline workout, something simple to remember and repeat without any equipment. This could be a one mile walk/jog/run, for example, where you see how long it takes you to walk/jog/run one mile, and repeat that as a test each month to see how much faster you can complete that mile. Or, it could be a bodyweight exercise test. Or, you could do both!

Example Three Minute Baseline Workout:

- Max push-ups (regular or modified from the wall, counter-top, or stairs): 1 minute

- Max squats: 1 minute

- Max seconds of forearm low plank: 1 minute

Do this work out on day one, and be sure to keep track of how many repetitions/seconds you can complete of each exercise in a one-minute period. Repeat this exact same workout once a month to see how many more repetitions/seconds you can perform for each move to gauge how much progress you have made. You will be shocked and thrilled to see how fast you can make progress if you keep up with physical activity on a consistent basis!

Keep track of each and every workout you complete in your Google Drive document or notebook. Write down how many sets and reps you completed, how much weight you used each time if applicable, how far you walked/jogged/ran each time, also if applicable. No matter what you choose to do, write it down. The goal is to do just a little bit better each time you work out than you did the time before. Using cellphone apps to help us track our movement and progress can also be a great tool. Ones that I've used are Couch to 5k Strava, Seconds Pro, RunKeeper, and Zombies, Run! (yes, I like to pretend I'm running from zombies now and then!) I'm sure there are boatloads of other awesome apps as well. Try out as many as you like (especially since most of them are free) to see which ones make you happy and fit into your exercise lifestyle. And ALWAYS remember to celebrate your efforts every time you complete a work out!

Breathing, Exercise Form, and Pre & Post-Exercise Nutrition:

One of the MOST IMPORTANT aspects of exercising is BREATHING. It sounds like a no-brainer, I know, but most people are naturally inclined to hold their breath while exercising. This is normal at first, but also harmful if we don't pay attention, because we are depriving our brains and muscles of the vital oxygen they need to keep us moving.

When doing weight-bearing exercise, whether bodyweight or with actual weights, get in the habit of training yourself to breathe in on the eccentric phase of the exercise, and out on the concentric phase. What that means is to exhale on exertion, or during the hardest part of the exercise. For example, when performing a push-up, the hardest part of the movement is pushing ourselves back up. It's pretty easy to lower down since gravity is giving us a pretty major assist, but when we push ourselves back up, we are on our own, and that's when we need to breathe out. The same goes for a pull-up; dropping down is easy, it's when we are pulling ourselves back up that is the hardest part and thus when we need to exhale. When performing a sit-up, it's when we are sitting back up that is the hardest part and again, when we need to exhale. This tip is important to consider, and is something that I've seen many clients struggle with in the beginning. Keep this tip in mind and you will always be able to easily figure out when to exhale!

The other extremely important factor to consider when doing weight-bearing exercises is learning and maintaining proper exercise form. You don't have to hire a trainer to learn this, although I will never advise against getting some professional assistance when trying to take things to the next level. There are endless *YouTube* videos (including my own!) that quickly explain and demonstrate the proper form for every single exercise that exists. It is absolutely worth the couple of minutes it takes to watch the videos before doing the exercise in order to protect our bodies from avoidable injuries.

When it comes to any exercise, it is always "quality over quantity!" Our bodies will always see more benefits from doing five perfect push-ups than doing ten with our pelvises dipping to the floor, and we are moving like snakes. Learning and maintaining proper form is the number-one way to avoid injury during weight-bearing exercises. No matter what position our body is in during an exercise, our head and neck should always be in a neutral position, or lined up with the spine.

For example, when doing a push-up, our gaze should be directed at the floor below, not up at something across the room or down at our feet. Think of placing a long stick up against your head, neck, and spine, and having the stick touch all three surfaces. This way, your head, neck, and spine will all remain in a straight line. Spinal integrity is no joke!

The last thing I want to mention is the importance of post-exercise nutrition. It is important to fuel our bodies with what they need so they can perform to their best abilities. This allows our bodies to maximize the effects of our workouts and to adapt and heal as quickly and efficiently as possible.

Post-exercise nutrition should come as soon as possible after the workout, ideally within 30 minutes. This is important because this meal will stop the catabolic effect of muscle breakdown and induce an anabolic effect of muscle adaptation and repair. After finishing a workout, think about eating somewhere around 15 grams of simple carbs (fruit) in addition to a lean protein; for example, a quality protein shake.

Anything high in fat (whether healthy or unhealthy fat) will slow down the digestion process, and we want the post-exercise nutrition to digest fast. So save the fats for earlier in the day or a little later, after the post-exercise nutrition has digested. As far as what to eat before a workout, what works best for each of us can be as varied as our entire nutritional lifestyles, depending on the time and type of workout.

There is no hard-and-fast rule that works for everyone. Some prefer exercising on an empty stomach, some do better with having some carbs and protein 30-60 minutes beforehand. Part of the experimentation process includes using that notebook and keeping track of how you feel and what your blood sugars reflect regarding what and when you eat, and using that information to figure out what works best for your body.

As someone who once hated exercise and thought I just wasn't made for it, I never would have thought exercise would become such an integral part of my identity. Now, it is literally, down to the core, part of who I am; and without it, I feel off physically, mentally, emotionally, and spiritually. This shift in perception and action not only helped me to drastically change the state of my health and my diabetes management, but it also changed the way I viewed my own abilities to conquer challenges of any kind, no matter what life threw at me.

Exercise showed me that the only person worth competing against is myself, to show myself that I am a little bit stronger each day. Once I figured out what I was capable of, I wanted to go further to see what else was possible. The feelings of freedom, confidence, and empowerment that come along with these changes are truly invaluable.

There are some great routines to follow in Part Three: Take Action that will help guide you in your exercise choices moving forward.

Exercise and Blood Sugars:

For those of us with diabetes, managing our blood sugars is usually the number-one challenge we have to work through when it comes to exercise. Believe me, I KNOW this can be a frustrating topic, and for many of us, can become the reason we choose not to work out at all. The main things I struggled with in the beginning (and occasionally still have to deal with, because hey, diabetes isn't going away!) and that ALL of my clients work to overcome are the exercise-induced lows and the mental/emotional fallout of feeling defeated when we've suited up and put forth the effort, only to go low during the activity and need to stop, or need to correct with unwanted carbs after we've just worked hard to burn those calories. I very deeply understand the frustrations of working out and then being forced to eat those calories we've just burned right back up, in the form of juice boxes and glucose tabs.

I have screamed and cried and kicked things over this very thing, more than once on my journey. However, just like any other challenge we face when it comes to living with diabetes, this is one that can be put in check more times than not. I'm not saying that there is a way to avoid lows all the time during or after exercise, but I am saying that we all have the ability to experiment and find a system that works best for us so we can have more wins than losses in this category.

Figuring out how our bodies will react to certain forms of exercise requires us to keep those notes in our workout notebook or in our online journal. For me, USUALLY when I do cardio, my blood sugar will begin to drop within 15 minutes; but when I do heavy weightlifting, it will begin to rise within 15 minutes. I say "usually" because as you and I both know, diabetes is not always predictable. However, more times than not, this is the pattern that my body follows, and it is up to each of us to figure out the patterns of our own bodies so we can feel confident when we exercise.

One thing that has been a helpful tool when it comes to managing blood sugars during exercise is suspending insulin delivery. Of course, this only works if you are on a pump. Out of my almost-25 years of living with diabetes, I've only had a pump for the past two-and-a-half years, so managing blood sugars without a pump during exercise is something with which I'm extremely familiar; and it can absolutely be done. However, if you are a pumper, the "suspend insulin delivery" function can be a huge difference-maker.

When I do cardio, I suspend insulin delivery for the entirety of the activity. When it comes to weightlifting, it's too variable to say.

Sometimes I need to inject a half-unit ahead of time; sometimes I don't need anything; and sometimes, once it's over, my blood sugar is rising so fast that I need a unit or more to get it back to normal. But with cardio, things are a bit more predictable.

I also actively plan to do cardio only when I have less than one unit of insulin on board, preferably none at all, but that's not always possible. If we have insulin on board (or if we've injected fast-acting insulin in the past couple of hours), it will likely affect our exercise routine. If there is no insulin on board, it is less likely that we will experience lows because without insulin and a properly functioning pancreas, it's much harder for a low blood sugar to occur.

That's the thing about exercise that I mentioned above: the effects on our blood sugars happen almost immediately. That's just one major reason it is so important to be comfortable adjusting our insulin needs on our own. When we exercise, we need less insulin overall. When we don't exercise, we need more insulin overall. Our insulin-to-carb ratios will likely also be affected right away, often making it so we need less insulin to cover the same amount of carbs as before we began exercising.

So if we are on MDI (manual daily injections), and we begin to exercise regularly, it is likely that we will need less basal insulin (long-acting insulin, Lantus, Levemir, etc.) and less fast-acting insulin pretty much right away. If we are pumpers, we will probably need to adjust (lower) our basal rates right away. How much less, I cannot say, as it will truly vary person-to-person, and I recommend talking to your endocrinologist, CDE, or other trusted team member to work out the specific numbers over time.

However, I strongly believe that becoming comfortable with adjusting our own insulin needs is a crucial aspect of feeling happy and confident regarding our diabetes management. Having a great healthcare team is important, and having them set a baseline for where to start is helpful and necessary. However, if we had a functioning pancreas, it wouldn't give us the same exact amounts of insulin at the same times each day.

Instead, it would give us different amounts of insulin based on what our daily activities consisted of. Some days we are more active than others; some days we eat more than others; and some days we are just plain old sick. All of these scenarios will require different amounts of insulin, and it is ultimately up to us to learn to understand and best anticipate those needs based on our experiences. Overall, this is why it is so beneficial to get into as regular a routine as possible, eating at as close to the same times as possible, and exercising on a consistent, predictable schedule so we can best anticipate our insulin needs.

15

SUPPORT

"Every time you smile at someone, it is an action of love, a gift to that person, a beautiful thing...Kind words can be short and easy to speak, but their echoes are truly endless."
-Mother Theresa

Before I was living in the Diabetes Dominator mentality, I remember (and I know my mom would back me up here) that I thought I could and should do everything on my own regarding my diabetes care. I thought that if I asked for help in any way, whether it was as simple as asking someone to grab me a juice box when I was low, or just sitting down and talking out my frustrations with someone, not even with the intention of having them fix anything, but just to get some of the built-up stress off my chest, that I was both showing weakness and burdening the other person.

Now I can tell you with 100% confidence that I WAS SO WRONG! Every time my mom would ask me what my blood sugar was or what I ate that day when I was in my teens, I would get mad at her. I'd tell her not to worry about it and that it wasn't her business, which she totally didn't deserve! Looking back (hindsight is always 20/20 right?), I now realize that not only was I hurting her feelings and making her feel helpless when she wanted nothing but to be helpful, but I was hurting myself as well.

Do you do this with anyone in your life? I know I'm not the only person who has dealt with this or continues to deal with these feelings and issues on a regular basis. I know how easy it is to default to the mindset of feeling like a burden, or convincing ourselves that people just don't understand what we are going through, so why even bother?

But I am here to tell you that I've been on both sides of this, and that choosing to stay in that mindset is not only perpetually damaging to ourselves, but also to those with whom we want to have good, functional relationships. Allowing people into our worlds, even if it is just through a conversation now and then, can be one of the most helpful experiences when it comes to managing life with diabetes. And although the other person might not truly understand exactly what we are going through, that will never change unless we give them some open and honest insights into our worlds.

As people with diabetes, sometimes getting the support we need means stepping (or leaping) outside our comfort zones. Sometimes our responsibilities go beyond our own self-care, to becoming a source of education, to being an advocate for what life is really like with diabetes, in order to quell the misconceptions that diabetes is easily manageable. That it's just as easy as counting carbs and getting insulin, and everything else just works itself out (which is unfortunately the way many people who don't live with diabetes think things go).

If we go about this with intention, having a specific outcome in mind (my intention is to educate, and my outcome is to grow closer to that person by sharing, for example), we in turn begin to welcome the support that we all so desperately need, whether we know it or not. The first and most important step is admitting that we need support, that we are not alone on Diabetes Island, that we are not a burden. It is a true sign of strength, not weakness, to reach out our hand and ask for the help we need.

Humans need support, it is built into our DNA. It's one thing to be proud, to have pride in being able to handle things on our own, but it is another thing entirely to allow that pride to fool us into believing that we don't need the support and compassion that only another human being can offer.

The good news is that there are a wide variety of support systems from which to choose. We have our in-person options, which could be made up of family, friends, co-workers, teachers, nurses, doctors, CDEs, nutritionists, dietitians, coaches, or pretty much anyone we talk to face-to-face. We have our virtual options, which could be made up of any of those listed above, via phone or Skype or Google Hangouts. Our support systems can also consist of the technology we use daily to keep ourselves on track (not that we can have two-sided conversations with these things, but they do support us!), such as our injections, pumps, meters and continuous glucose monitors, and online tools. These can include www.myfitnesspal.com, where we track our food intakes, or Google

Drive documents, which are free and allow us to create categories that fit our specific daily tracking needs that we can check off each day to keep ourselves on-track.

All of this online talk is leading me to what might be the most valuable support system of all, the system that allowed me to feel like I was part of a team for the first time in my life years ago, the support system that gave me the confidence I needed to finally write this book, and to finally know that I'm not alone living with diabetes. The support system that is there 24/7/365, without judgement (for the most part; because no matter where we go, people are people, and there are always going to be some rude people out there, but they are for sure the minority), always accepting me with open arms, and that will do the same for you. A support system where you can choose to remain anonymous for as long as you like and still experience deep, profound connections. The one, the only…

Diabetes Online Community (DOC for short)

The diabetes online community is an incredible place. A place that any of us can go anytime to find the support we need. A place with a seemingly endless variety of support systems that allow us to decide where we feel comfortable and where we fit in. A place that, in reality, is still in its beginning stages, since it's really no more than 15-or-so years old and it's growing more and more every day.

A place where all voices are welcome and valued and appreciated because everyone's diabetes experience is just a little different (As Bennet Dunlap always says, and is also the name of his blog, Your Diabetes May Vary), even though we all experience much of the same thing. Where we can be ourselves without having to explain our diabetes, because, well, everyone either has it themselves or loves someone who does. The DOC really is a magical place where diabetes is the norm, and that in itself is a welcome change to the reality of day-to-day life in the "real world," where we often have to explain something about our diabetes management to someone who isn't familiar with it (which is totally okay, but it's so nice when everyone just "gets it").

Whether we want to read a blog or an article on the topic of something with which we are currently struggling, written by a person with diabetes; watch an interview between two people living with diabetes, just so we can relate to the topic of conversation; or we want to live-chat with someone else who has diabetes and really just "gets it" no matter what we say, the DOC has our backs.

Very often when I tell fellow people with diabetes about the DOC who aren't actively involved in it already, the first thing they ask me is where they can find it, which is a very good question. It can be found all over the internet, but there is no "official" page that lists all of the amazing sites to check out in order to find the information for which we are searching. For now, I decided to start a page at **www.diabetesoc.com,** where I've just begun to compile a list of as many of these blogs, articles, forums, *YouTube* channels, and other resources, for easier navigation of this vast and awesome community of amazingness. I will continually add to this site forever, and welcome any suggestions for resources that should be added. If you have any suggestions, email me at Coach@diabetesdominator.com, and we can continue to build this DOC homepage, as it were, together!

And that's pretty much the best thing about the DOC: it shows us that we are not alone, even though many of us (including me) have spent countless years feeling like we are taking on this disease and all of the emotional tolls that it takes on our lives by ourselves, which is an incredibly heavy burden to bear. It allows us to finally connect with our brothers and sisters and build our own tribes. It allows us to understand, accept, and finally embrace that we are all in this diabetes thing together, and we are so much stronger (and happier and more at peace and capable of fighting back) as a team than we could ever be alone.

The bottom line of the support section is that without being willing to reach out for and accept consistent support, we will ultimately continue to feel alone. This is not only true for those of us living with diabetes, but also for any human being who wants to achieve anything in life. Great achievements are not reached alone.

For example, Olympic skier and type 1 diabetic Kris Freeman would have never been an Olympic skier without constant support from his coaches, family, friends, doctors, his pump and his CGM, and his consistent tracking of his food intake, exercise regimen, and blood sugar levels. He is the only person we see out there actually skiing, but he certainly couldn't have gotten to the slopes alone. My advice is that no matter what might be holding you back from getting some support, which is most likely your own mentality or ideas about what reaching out for support means (as was the case for me for so long), is to simply let it go.

We must get over our imagined fears of burdening those who care for us, and the fact that we've convinced ourselves that we are strong enough to do everything alone...no one is! Living with a chronic disease is not a burden that is meant to be carried alone...ever. The sooner we are able to let go of our old beliefs that aren't serving our wellbeing, the sooner we will be on the path to living the quality of life we desire.

Taking the DOC from Online to In-Person: The Enriching and Uplifting Experience of Attending Diabetes Conferences and Volunteering

As amazing as the DOC is, there is nothing like taking the online experience to real life. Hugs galore. Love and acceptance. Friends for life. I can't say enough good things about what transformations occur when we surround ourselves with our like-minded peers. For me, I never went to diabetes camp as a child, so every time I go to a diabetes conference, it's kind of like what I imagine camp would've been like. I get to see all of my friends and we get to hang out, learn, grow, and play together. There are countless conferences to attend all over the USA and internationally as well. Here are a few that I highly recommend!

The Diabetes UnConference, http://diabetesunconference.com

This event is unlike any other diabetes conference I have ever had the pleasure of attending. The UnConfernece is the first of its kind, in that it is a peer-to-peer experience, where people with all types of diabetes come together as one big family to learn from and support each other. It was created via the love and passion of an amazing fellow T1D, Christel Marchand Aprigliano. The following description is taken from the UnConference website: "An 'unconference' allows participants to create and moderate the agenda, allowing for a wide variety of topics and viewpoints that might never be covered in a traditional conference. Using various sharing methods that focus on drawing out responses from all attendees, those in the room learn from each other in a peer-to-peer environment." I can't recommend attending the UnConference highly enough, any time you get a chance!

Children with Diabetes Friends for Life Conference, http://www.childrenwithdiabetes.com/activities/

This conference was created 16 years ago by a mom of a type 1 child, who, more than anything else, was looking for other families living with diabetes to hang out with. Laura Billetdeaux simply wanted to go to Disney World with her type 1 son and the rest of their family; and in the process, "accidentally" created one of the longest running conferences for people living with diabetes and their families to come together to learn and have a ton of fun. Conference-goers get to attend educational sessions and get cutting-edge diabetes management ideas. We get to participate in discussion groups, share our stories, and help motivate and support others who walk in similar shoes. We get to see toddlers and teens; college students and professionals; young parents and grandparents; and new and practiced diabetes clinicians make new and lifelong friendships. This is a conference you won't ever forget!

MasterLab via Diabetes Advocates/Diabetes Hands Foundation, http://diabetesadvocates.org/masterlab

For anyone who is interested in learning how easy it is to raise awareness (and your voice) for diabetes advocacy, attend this program. While held in the same space as the Friends for Life's conference, it's a separate conference. Last year's program was amazing! I know this first-hand, as I was lucky enough to win a scholarship to attend, and I can't wait to go back next year.

Taking Control of Your Diabetes (TCOYD), https://tcoyd.org/

TCOYD has a mission statement that I couldn't love or agree with more, both as a person with diabetes and a person who helps others who live with diabetes find their path to a sustainable healthy lifestyle. The mission statement reads: "Guided by the belief that every person with diabetes has the right to live a healthy, happy, and productive life, Taking Control of Your Diabetes educates and motivates people with diabetes to take a more active role in their condition and provides innovative and integrative continuing diabetes education to medical professionals caring for people with diabetes." TCOYD was created by Dr. Steven Edelman, who has been living with diabetes himself for over four decades. TCOYD puts on a wide variety of conferences and events every year, and attending any of them is sure to be an incredibly uplifting and educational experience that I highly recommend.

Volunteering is Where It's At

Volunteering our time for a cause that is close to our hearts is so overwhelmingly fulfilling. The American Diabetes Association gave me the opportunity to volunteer at various Boys' and Girls' clubs and YMCAs, teaching kids about type 2 diabetes prevention and nutrition, and I am forever grateful for that opportunity. There are endless ways that anyone can lend a hand and volunteer their time to help support diabetes awareness.

Both the American Diabetes Association and the Juvenile Diabetes Research Foundation (JDRF) have local chapters that need and appreciate any help you are willing to give. And there is just no way to describe the fulfillment we get when we give of ourselves in order to serve others. When we give our precious time and attention to benefit the greater good of a cause we believe in, it fills our hearts with joy! Volunteering is the perfect way to support ourselves and others at the same time.

Diabetes Advocacy: Why Every Single One of Our Voices Matter, How to Very Easily Make a Difference, and Why We Are Stronger When We Are Not Separated by Types

"Advocacy" is defined by Merriam-Webster as "public support for or recommendation of a particular cause or policy," or "the act or process of supporting a cause or proposal." Being a diabetes advocate, or advocating for diabetes awareness in any way that is helpful to our community, is important and necessary; and the more people who participate, the more positive changes we will see over time. Diabetes advocacy comes in many shapes and forms, and they all add value to each of us individually, and to our community as a whole.

From writing a blog or article, to posting information on social media, to having a simple conversation with someone we meet in line at the supermarket or at our local pharmacy, there are many ways in which we can all be diabetes advocates. I see advocacy as the act of using our voices to help educate, spread awareness, and/or offer compassion or empathy to both ourselves and others who need any or all of these things when it comes to all aspects of living with diabetes.

Another great thing about diabetes advocacy is that you don't have to have diabetes yourself to be an effective diabetes advocate; you just have to have the facts straight and be willing to spread awareness and knowledge to others. When we live with diabetes every day or love someone who does, it can be easy to lose sight of the fact that most of the general public truly has no real idea of what diabetes is all about, or what goes into managing such a time-consuming disease. Many people also don't know critical information like the signs and symptoms of diabetes, which are crucial for early detection and, in many cases, the ability to save that person's life.

And we all know that so many people just don't know what to say (or not say) or how to react when interacting with someone with diabetes when they see us check our blood sugar or go to inject, for example. I am barely scratching the surface here regarding the almost-infinite ways in which we can advocate for diabetes awareness. Each person who we are able to enlighten, even just the slightest bit, now possesses that knowledge and, even more importantly, now has the ability to pass it on to someone else.

The more people who know what diabetes is really about, the better. Just to be clear, I'm not being naïve here. I don't think the issues surrounding the misconceptions or untruths about diabetes will be fixed overnight, or even anytime in the immediate future. But I do believe that the more of us who speak-up in a non-confrontational manner– not fueled by anger, but by the true desire to spread awareness–the more that people will know and want to spread the facts instead of the slew of current perpetuated untruths.

The fact is that there are around 30 million of us with diabetes in the USA, and about 387 million of us worldwide, and the numbers are growing steadily. Although ours isn't a team that anyone asks to join, we are nonetheless a growing team of incredibly amazing human beings, all with the power to advocate for the awareness of our disease and to help stop the spread of sheer ignorance to simple facts. And we will always be stronger when we stick together and unite our voices for the greater good of our community, versus shouting from the rooftops on our own. United we stand, divided we fall. The more we educate about how eating too much sugar isn't what causes type 1 diabetes and isn't the only factor involved in the development of type 2 diabetes, for example, slowly but surely, people will learn the facts.

These times, although I know they can be extremely trying and difficult not to take personally, are some of the most golden opportunities to advocate, educate, and spread the correct information so that, slowly, we can help eradicate these often hurtful misconceptions. These are the times to reach out to our DOC and ask for other voices to join us in advocating for the truth. Trust me, I know and feel how much it hurts to be blamed for our condition. I've been through it many times over the past 24 years.

But one thing I've found to remain true is that freaking out with violent rage and fighting back with intense vitriol and hate never helps the situation. And further, reacting in that way often exacerbates things to a point where we look like the ones who are in the wrong, when really we are just trying to defend ourselves and the truth. When this happens, it takes the focus completely off of the issue at hand, which is our trying to spread facts and make information about diabetes more common knowledge.

Instead, a personal fight ensues between each of us as individuals against whoever spread the mistruth in the first place.

This leads to personal attacks that hold no bearing and fighting over issues that were never part of the original argument; both of which get us, as a community, no further than we were before it all started. It takes a big person to remain calm in the face of hurt, misinformation, and the need to defend something as hugely personal as living with diabetes every single day or loving someone who does. But, in my opinion, it is the only way we will ever begin to put a dent in this ongoing issue.

> *"Education is the most powerful weapon which you can use to change the world."*
> -Nelson Mandela

I will never say that this is or will be an easy journey, but I will say that if we are able to keep our peers in mind each time the opportunity arises to spread the truth, and know that we are going to bat not only for ourselves, but also for millions of our brothers and sisters, it might be just a tiny bit easier to keep our cool so we don't end up looking crazy (trust me, I've been that crazy person one too many times!) And, in truth, I know we're not being crazy. I know we are passionate about making it clear that we are not to blame for our disease, that we are human beings living with a chronic illness, and we have every right to be upset.

But sometimes in ongoing "wars" of sorts, it pays off in the long run to be the more diplomatic party and let the other side "talk themselves out," so to speak. That way, we are collectively the calm, cool, educated party that is simply spreading facts, rather than adding fuel to an already much too gassed-up fire. Anyone who knows me knows that I am not a docile person. People who know me well know that I say what I feel, am a strongly passionate person, and will always defend my brothers and sisters.

I spent many years of my life full of unrelenting anger and rage, and I've been called the "B" word more times than I can count. However, through years of self-reflection and intense, intentional personal development, I've learned that there is a fine line between passionate and psychotic; and I know this because it is a line that I've crossed many times before. Through personal experience, I've learned that being able to recognize and be aware and mindful of when this might have a chance of happening, can be the deciding factor in whether or not we achieve the outcome we are truly after. It is a very tough thing to master, especially when it comes to a subject we are all rightfully passionate about, but when we do, we will find that we will make more headway for our cause than we ever imagined possible.

Diabetes Patient Advocacy Coalition (DPAC): www.diabetespac.org

There is another hugely important way that we can advocate for diabetes. A way that doesn't involve any arguing, blogging, or social media involvement if we don't want there to be. A way that simply requires us to use our computers to reach out to the political powers that be, so we can get diabetes-related issues brought to the forefront, in front of the eyes of those who have the power to change or enact new laws.

Things like the quality of blood glucose meter accuracy, which we use to determine our insulin dosing, our safety as patients in care facilities, rights that those of us living with diabetes have as patients, or making sure we have access to the supplies we need to live healthy lives. If you are thinking that just one voice doesn't really matter, please believe me and know that every single voice does matter, and that DPAC has made it foolproof for us, as a community of 30 million-strong in the United States, to speak-up together.

They have made it possible for us to come together as a united team so that our issues get the attention they deserve–the issues that have been seriously lacking attention for too many years now. I will never try to force you to do something, as I believe that meaningful action needs to be taken by choice, BUT this is the one and only exception. If you have a computer, cellphone, or any internet access at all, and you don't take this action, you are actively choosing not to use the easiest and least labor-intensive avenue for advocating for our team, and for yourself.

You are choosing not to stand up for yourself and your rights as a human being living with diabetes, or who loves someone living with diabetes. No pressure! And I promise you that I wouldn't be so adamant about this if it wasn't so incredibly, ridiculously easy to do. It can literally be done in a matter of five minutes or less.

The way things change in politics involves how many times our senators and congressmen see our issues come across their desks. DPAC has created a way for us to speak directly to our local representatives by simply putting in our zip codes, typing in our names, and hitting "submit." No kidding. No gimmicks. And major changes have already begun to come about from people taking action through the platform that this incredible non-profit organization has created for us as patients.

So this is the one and only time I will beg of you, PLEASE go to **www.diabetespac.org,** follow the instructions, and let your voice be heard as it deserves to; share this information freely on social media and otherwise, and encourage others to do the same whether they have diabetes or not. And just so you know, DPAC isn't just some faceless organization. DPAC was co-founded and is run by patients with diabetes: Bennet Dunlap and Christel Marchand Aprigliano, both of whom I am blessed to know personally, so I can vouch for their selflessness when it comes to serving our incredible diabetes community. Thank you for stepping up. We all need you…we all need each other!

Peer Diabetes Advocacy

I'm working on a special peer diabetes advocacy project and I'd love to have you along for the ride. If you'd like more information and to stay updated on the progress of this project, sign up at **peerdiabetes.org.**

Mending the Divide Between Types

When it comes to diabetes, we all know that, medically speaking, there are different types. We have type 1, type 2, LADA, MODY, gestational, pre-diabetes, and with the rate at which medical science is making new discoveries about how our bodies work, there could be five other types by the time this book comes out. However, in the long run, none of that matters one tiny bit when it comes to advocating for our rights as patients and getting laws changed in our favor.

We all need our medications to live and thrive. We all need access to safe and quality products and services. We all deserve to be treated as human beings, not just walking chronic illnesses, and we've all struggled with one or more of these issues before, and most likely will again.

Are there medical differences between us as types? Sure. But the bottom line is, if we choose to spend time fighting amongst ourselves about not wanting to be categorized as one type or another, all of that effort goes to waste, and we are no better off than before. If we don't come together, nothing is going to get done to further our patient rights, and we all essentially have the same needs that aren't being met.

Here's the kicker: I spent a good amount of time scouring the internet, and couldn't find another disease that affected nearly as many people, not even by a longshot. But the thing is, other diseases get MUCH MORE legislative attention. We have the power as a team, as a community, to band together and change our standing in the legislative rankings.

We are all human beings who didn't ask for this burden, no matter what type of diabetes we have, and when things change for the better for one type, all other types benefit in some way or another. Type 1s are now using medications that were previously thought to only be effective for type 2s, and vice versa. All types benefit from CGMs, and all types use pumps, syringes, and insulin. Things are changing all the time, and the more effort we put into getting the attention we need as a whole, the better off every single one of us will be. I don't care what type you are. You are all my peers, part of my diabetes team, my diabetes family. We will always be stronger when we stick together and have each other's backs.

Building Our Diabetes Care Team and Learning to Trust Our Instincts

***Reminder: I am not a medical doctor. Any changes you make to your medications should be discussed with your healthcare team first.

Over my 24+ years of living with diabetes, I have had more than a few visits with various endocrinologists; many of whom, let's just say, didn't see things the way I did. I am very fortunate to now have an endocrinologist who I like, but it did take some trial and error to find her. Unfortunately, diabetes is not a "by-the-books" disease, and unless you live with it yourself day-to-day or care for someone who lives with it day-to-day, it is difficult (some might say impossible) to understand the intricacies of daily life with this disease, and to best advise people on how to proceed.

Please don't misunderstand me here and stop seeing your endocrinologist! Just know that you have rights as a patient, and that, just like dealing with any other service provider, we have the right to seek out a new doctor if the one we have isn't providing us with an experience that we feel satisfied with.

We must also be aware that what they recommend is not always the end-all-be-all, and if what they are telling us doesn't seem logical or right for us, then it's most likely not. Every person with diabetes has different needs and has a different experience physically, mentally, and emotionally. This is something our doctors must recognize, and also ultimately understand that they are not treating a disease, but rather a person. Each patient is a uniquely individual human being who has the right to be heard and whose opinions need to be valued and taken into consideration when making recommendations about how to proceed in all aspects of diabetes management.

Although our medical care team is very much necessary and beneficial, diabetes is a disease whose management is 99% in our hands. The doctor's portion of our support systems can only truly contribute to our wellness in small increments, in the form of advice here and there to help us find our best management practices. The day-to-day care and the moment-to-moment decisions, however, are up to us. If we remain in the mindset that our doctors can totally manage our diabetes for us, we will eventually realize that isn't a realistic option.

Using the Valuable Tools We Have to Our Advantage

Checking our blood sugar, and checking it OFTEN is the most valuable tool we have to help us understand what is going on inside of our bodies, and is also the best way we can support any changes and new habits we choose to create. Before I was lucky enough to get a Dexcom continuous glucose monitor (CGM) about three years ago, I checked my blood sugar an average of 12-16 times a day, my goal being to check once every hour I was awake. I had to tell my doctor that I needed to check that often, and (somewhat) politely insist that she write the prescription for test strips to reflect my need to test that often, since she thought this was excessive at first until I explained my motives to take the best possible care of myself. It is my genuine hope that sometime in the near future, CGMs will be mandatory medical equipment that are prescribed to every person with diabetes. But until then, we have to be our own biggest advocates and supporters because, unfortunately, the DOC can't come to our doctor's appointments with us (yet).

Those of us living with diabetes know that our blood sugars can wildly fluctuate in a matter of minutes, and this is something that doctors must take into consideration when recommending how often we check our blood sugar levels. If we are checking our blood sugars any less than ten times a day and have the supplies necessary to do so, we are lacking incredibly valuable information that is key to our abilities to thrive. The tools we have are only helpful if we choose to use them.

It is impossible to make informed decisions about correcting highs or treating lows if we don't know the numbers. Again, this is an example of not being able to manage what we don't measure. I know that many doctors recommend checking 3-5 times a day, basically before and after meals, which, in my opinion, is insane if we really want to know what is going on with our health.

I've learned this over the years, as I have heard this from the majority my clients when I ask them how many times a day they are checking. Guesswork is not a safe or healthy way to determine diabetes management practices. If we have enough supplies and are able to measure and track our blood sugar levels at any given moment, but don't do so because our doctor recommended differently, or because we've convinced ourselves that it's too much of a hassle, or something along those lines, we are doing ourselves a great disservice.

We all know that checking our blood sugar takes less than one minute, on average, so time and ease aren't deterring factors for most of us. A massive part of the learning and growing process when it comes to diabetes management is learning to trust our instincts, logic, and common sense. We must be willing to admit that we might have been wrong about the choices we were making in the past, and that being wrong is completely okay and part of being human. I have been wrong so many times in the past and will continue to do so in the future, I'm sure; but it was my willingness to finally admit it that allowed me to make changes and make progress where I was otherwise stuck for so long.

I have recently had the immense pleasure and luxury of incorporating a Dexcom CGM into my life (it has been about three years so far), and it has largely changed the quality of my health and the quality of my life. I went 22 out of my almost-25 years with diabetes without it, so it is absolutely possible to be highly successful without one. However, the freedom and power of knowing what my blood sugar is at any given moment, and knowing whether it is trending up, down, or staying steady at the click of a button is nothing short of outstanding.

The Dexcom (they are not paying me to say this; I just love it so much!) allows me to feel an even higher level of confidence and liberation, particularly while exercising and sleeping. The trend arrows allow the user to make corrections before getting too high or too low, which is invaluable. If you have the undeniably crappy issue of insurance's lack of coverage for it (which is currently the case for everyone over the age of 65), or you don't have insurance at all, it is still worthwhile to contact Dexcom (their customer support is stellar) to see if there are any other options, so you have all the information before making any decisions.

Like Wayne Gretzky says, "You miss 100% of the shots you don't take." This is worth a phone call. Even if it doesn't pan out immediately, there is no need to get discouraged. Things are rapidly changing in the world of diabetes technology, and there will very likely be more affordable options in the near future.

Please visit diabetesdominator.com/bookresources and view some of my CGM readouts to see some examples of the valuable information the Dexcom offers.

For 23 of my almost 25 years of living with diabetes, I happily and successfully used manual daily injections. However, about six months after introducing the Dexcom into my life, I decided to give a pump a try…I like to experiment. However, the only way I was willing to do that was if the pump was tubeless, and Omnipod provided me with an amazing way to experience what life with a pump is like. Once I began using the Omnipod, I haven't looked back. This is a very personal decision, and I strongly believe that, much like a nutritional lifestyle, each individual must decide what works best for them.

For me, I can say that without a doubt, using the Omnipod and the Dexcom together allowed me to lower my A1c to the lowest it's ever been in my almost 25 years of living with diabetes. I love the Omnipod, and the fact that I change my site every three days, and never think about injecting at all in between. I love the data it provides me—I no longer have to worry about whether or not I bolused for a meal since I can just bring up my history on the PDM and verify. Again, this is just my experience, and I know lots of people who are wildly successful in their diabetes management with other pumps and using MDI. I'm just giving my two cents!

As far as meters go, I have been using a OneTouch UltraMini for around 7 years now. I like it because it's really small, and if I want to take it out of the case and put it in a small purse it is easily transportable. It also helps that my insurance company covers the test strips. They have different colors to choose from, and overall I've personally found that the accuracy is usually pretty spot on.

My OneTouch UltraMini and my Dexcom are within 10 mg/dl of each other I'd say about 85% of the time or more. So for what it's worth, I like my OneTouch very much, and choose to use it over the meter that is built into my Omnipod. I'm not saying that the FreeStyle meter that's built into the Omnipod isn't great and reliable as well, I've just never personally tested it to find out for myself so I can't offer a valid opinion on the matter.

The Human Experience, Processing Our Stories, and Supporting Diabetes So it can Support Us

The best way to stay on track is to focus and concentrate on what is going right and why. And when something is off, instead of getting angry or discouraged, ask why it might be happening, and choose to make adjustments instead of giving up. I am so grateful that we live in a time where we have the tools and the freedoms to experiment with and find what works best for us individually.

Replacing the word "failure" with "experience" not only changes our mindset and our emotional responses to a much more progress-oriented direction, but it leaves us with less disappointment, heartache, and self-blame as well. As human beings, we are all walking science experiments, and there is no scientist better equipped at understanding our needs than ourselves. The context in which we think about our diabetes greatly affects the relationship we have with it, and being aware of this can be a game-changer. I used to think that my diabetes was a curse, a punishment, and I treated it as such. I fought with it, screamed at it, cursed at it, and hated it. When I began changing my mind about what was and was not possible for my life with diabetes, however, I began changing the context in which I viewed my relationship with diabetes.

Now, I actively choose to compare the way I treat my diabetes to the way I treat my pets that I love and care for very deeply. They are a part of my life, and I must nurture them and treat them with love and care to see them thrive. I must make sure they have what they need to live well every single day.

I never do anything before making sure my diabetes is in a safe place and well taken care of. The more love and support I show it, the better our relationship becomes. Putting diabetes into such loving terms can be difficult, as we all know it isn't a burden we chose to bear, and we didn't do anything to deserve all of the effort and hard work that goes into thriving with diabetes. However, our realities are truly shaped by the way we react to the things we experience.

I've attended many personal development events and seminars in my life. Recently, I heard Dr. Joan Rosenberg, who is a highly regarded doctor, expert psychologist, master clinician, trainer, and consultant, put the human grieving process into a context that made so much sense to me that I began crying when I related it to my relationship with diabetes. We all have our own ways of processing our personal stories–the stories we tell ourselves about who we are.

Living with diabetes requires a grieving process, in part because we deal with perceived losses every single day. But at the end of the day, we all must process our own stories and grieve our own human experiences; sometimes something so simple can be so incredibly profound. According to Dr. Rosenberg, there are five elements to that grieving process:

1. We grieve something we got and didn't deserve. (Diabetes!)
2. We grieve something we deserved but didn't get. (A life without diabetes!)
3. We grieve something that never was. (For some of us, a life without diabetes!)
4. We grieve something that isn't happening now that may have been happening before. (For some of us, a life without diabetes!)
5. We grieve something that may never be. (A life without diabetes!)

These things can be applied to all aspects of life (death of loved ones, lost love, etc.), but for the sake of this book, I'm keeping it all in the context of diabetes. Many of us (including myself) are still grieving our experiences with diabetes in one or more of these contexts. Just seeing it put so simply was a deeply moving moment for me, in a seminar where 150 other people were relating these steps to their own experiences.

How many of us feel like diabetes is a burden we didn't choose to bear, and one we don't deserve? Nobody wants to be blamed for their unsolicited burden, and becoming aware of and processing our stories through this simple five-step process can offer insights that we may not have previously been able to identify on our own.

Awareness and Preparedness

A bit of foresight and preparing ahead can lessen the burden of an already annoying or stressful situation. Having a game plan for unexpected situations is crucial, and so is expecting the unexpected. Of course, we can't predict the future, but we can be prepared for any number of occasions with just a little bit of ACTION. There are several scenarios that may happen at unexpected times, for which it is important to be prepared when living with diabetes. Using the simple, everyday tools we have at our disposal, like (recurring) reminders and alarms in our cellphones, can be the key to being ready for (almost) anything.

Running out of medications and supplies: If you do have health insurance and it is an option, choosing a three-month supply of medication and supplies through a prescription mail delivery service can be a game-changer. If you can choose this option and also go on automatic refill, even better. It still remains up to us to be proactive and tell our doctors what we need, including that we need to check our blood sugars 15 times a day. I know that might sound like a lot, but most of us are awake for 16 or more hours each day, and in order to best manage our blood sugars, we need to check about once an hour.

Any doctor who is a decent human being and a supportive member of our diabetes care team should understand our desire to take the best care of our health as is possible. And maybe the insurance won't cover it, but we won't know unless we try. Building a team of professionals who are on our sides is one of the most important things we can do. We must be proactive in building our team—a good team won't just fall into our lives!

Another option is going to local free-clinics. Sometimes when we are candid and tell them we have diabetes and can't afford certain supplies, they will give us some samples to hold us over, or help in some other way. The same goes for our endocrinologists or PCPs. Tell them you are having trouble, and more times than not, they will have free samples of insulin and test strips that they can offer you to help supplement your lack of supplies.

Many of the pharmaceutical companies that make our insulin also offer assistance programs if we contact them. My point here is that the squeaky wheel gets the oil! Don't be afraid or too proud to speak-up if you don't have the supplies you need; speak-up and speak often!

There is a great app called **HelpAround** that was specifically designed to allow people with diabetes to connect with others in their surrounding areas who might be able to offer assistance when certain supplies are needed. Another step we can take in order to get the supplies we need outside of insurance companies is to join any number of diabetes social media groups, specifically on *Facebook*, where there are countless groups made for people with diabetes, where we can help others in need of supplies and also barter/trade supplies with others who may need something we have.

I have listed some of these groups on **www.diabetesoc.com.** While in these closed groups, I see lots of people sharing information; but more, they are willing to give away or sell for just the cost of shipping all varieties of diabetes necessities. You can post what it is you are looking for and very often, people will kindly reach out to help if they can.

Now, I can see where you might be worried that these supplies might not be safe to use since they are not coming directly from the pharmacy. Here is where I say that common sense is always the best way to handle these types of situations. If you get medications or supplies from someone, make sure to check to see if they have been opened or if they are expired. Don't use products that have been opened, and make sure no seals are broken. If you have any doubts, don't use it. In the five plus years I have been in these groups, the people have been consistently kind and have had a kindred spirit with each other, as we are all going through the same issues.

When I was 19 years old, lasting into my 20s, I went through a dark period of years where I didn't have health insurance. I swallowed my pride and went to the local welfare office to see if I could get any assistance with my medical supplies, as I couldn't afford the things I needed to live. After waiting hours to speak to someone, I was informed that since I had a job (I was a waitress and a student) and didn't have any children, welfare couldn't offer me any assistance.

I left the office in a tearful rage, once again sure that I was being punished for some unknown horror I must have committed in a past life. I eventually took a job where I could get insurance as soon as possible (which for a couple of years was as a bartender in a hotel, and the insurance was really poor, and I had to fight tooth and nail for every prescription I got filled). In that time when I had no insurance, I amassed an exorbitant amount of credit card debt paying for my supplies.

And another real truth about how diabetes has affected my life is the quickness with which my husband and I chose to get married. I met my husband in August of 2006, and we got married in August of 2007. Granted, we loved each other intensely and were committed to spending our lives together, but one of the biggest factors that made us decide to get married ASAP was that he had insurance through his job and I desperately needed it. Navigating diabetes without insurance is no joke, and I feel the pain of those who suffer with this reality every day. The good thing is that there are many more options now than there were back then, as long as we are willing to take action and look into what is available for us.

Traveling and Flying with a Pump and/or CGM: Traveling the world and experiencing different cultures and ways of life is one of my biggest passions and favorite things to do, so I wasn't about to let having diabetes hinder my ability to travel, and neither should you! Personally, I haven't had too many issues while traveling with a giant bag of medical supplies, other than the occasional bag search, hand swipe, and once or twice being taken into a room and patted down by female TSA agents.

Sure, it's a hassle, but I take it for what it is and nothing more. Most of the agents are just doing their jobs and aren't trying to aggravate us, although there is, of course, always a chance of running into a miserable person anywhere. It's not a personal attack, and most times, it's no problem at all. Sometimes it even gives us a chance to have a friendly conversation with the agents and educate them about pumps and/or CGMs so they are better informed the next time they encounter one.

Having a note from a doctor explaining our need to carry our supplies can be helpful in situations like that, but for me, it's never been a necessity. If you wear a pump or a CGM, it is recommended that you don't go through the X-ray scanner. Instead, request a manual pat-down, which is totally fine and has never been an issue for me. I personally have gone through the X-ray scanner many times and have never had a problem with my pump or CGM afterwards.

I simply tell the agent that I'm wearing an insulin pump and a continuous glucose monitor. They ask me to touch both the CGM and the pump, and then they swab my hands with a little cloth and run the cloth through a machine to make sure there aren't any bomb-related materials on my hands. The whole process usually takes under three minutes.

Being prepared for and aware of what to expect can make all the difference in our travel experiences. Being proactive versus reactive can change the outcome of any experience. I highly recommend reading the following article if you are traveling with a pump that has tubing (any pump other than Omnipod); very important and helpful info!

http://asweetlife.org/feature/what-you-should-know-about-flying-with-an-insulin-pump/

Sex: This is a subject that doesn't get nearly enough (if any at all) coverage when it comes to how it factors into living with diabetes. Most doctors won't mention it, mainly because they don't know there's anything to mention in the first place. In reality, they couldn't know that there was anything to address unless they themselves had diabetes or were intimate on a regular basis with someone who did, or if they were told by a patient.

If you are a child/teen or a parent of a child/teen who is not sexually active, consider this information valuable knowledge that can be stored away and used at a later time. Even though it might feel awkward to discuss, I promise that you and your child will be better off knowing this stuff ahead of time; I certainly wish I had! Sex can (and often does) cause rapid (and I mean RAPID) fluctuations in blood sugar levels, usually in the way of low blood sugars.

And let me tell you, there is nothing sexier than getting insanely dizzy, confused, disoriented, and nauseous all of a sudden while in the throes of passion, and needing to tell your partner you have to stop and drink a juice box or eat glucose tabs, and then wait 15 minutes until you start feeling human again. Sounds hot, right? Just kidding. Trust me, it's not; it's actually pretty terrible.

My advice is, again, to take actions to be prepared ahead of time. Check your blood sugar right beforehand (if possible), and keep a juice box within arm's reach. Also, it's super important to inform your partner that you have diabetes and that something like this could happen. Overall, I hope that if you are at that level of intimacy with someone, that the person will already be aware of your diabetes. And if they don't already know, they will definitely find out if your blood sugar drops, and that's not the best time for delivering the news.

Illness and Menstruation: I'm linking these two topics together because the actions that need to be taken in both scenarios are pretty much the same, and the results that they each have on our diabetes are also generally the same. Menstruation is a very real part of a female's life that happens every single month, and, for many of us, can actually make us feel much worse than having a common cold. When we get sick (or get our period) and we have diabetes, it can be a wild ride on the blood sugar roller-coaster, with no real rhyme, reason, or patterns to be found. Here are some important actions to take as soon as you realize you are getting sick or that time of the month is approaching, in order to mitigate those blood sugar fluctuations as much as possible (if at all possible; sometimes these things work and make a real difference, and sometimes not so much).

Being properly hydrated can make a huge difference. Drinking at least half our bodyweight in ounces, even adding 20-30 extra ounces of water, is a must in these scenarios. Our aim is to keep a steady stream of filtration going on to help our bodies eliminate toxins that are being released into the bloodstream. Choosing whole, nutrient-dense foods around this time (although that might not be what we are craving) as much as possible is also super helpful. The more vegetables and fruits we can eat, the better. Eating foods that cleanse our bodies instead of clogging our already compromised systems allow our bodies to concentrate on kicking out that illness or easing up on menstrual symptoms.

For us ladies, taking a Vitamin B and a Vitamin C supplement for seven days prior to the start of our cycles, especially if we are not eating a lot of fruits and vegetables, can also make a big difference. These supplements would also be helpful to take during times of having a cold. Another helpful action is to set alarms to check our blood sugars every 1-2 hours to best stay on top of fighting those big fluctuations, as they can and do happen more often when the body is trying to fight off any kind of illness or is dealing with hormonal fluctuations.

And as we know, the more our blood sugars are in a healthy range, the better we will feel, not only in general, but especially when we are under the weather. Don't even get me started on having high blood sugars while being sick; it's an even more horrible feeling than usual! Try to avoid it from happening as much as possible by being proactive. Even if it still fluctuates (and it most likely will), don't give up. Give yourself massive props for stepping up and being incredibly strong and doing what most others won't. Even if others don't see them, our struggles shape our character, and that shows through in all that we do in life.

16

BODY SYSTEMS

"Well done is better than well said."
-Benjamin Franklin

In this section, I am only going to cover two topics.
However, these are the two most important functions that our bodies
need to perform every single day. These two aspects of our lives
massively affect our health and wellness in every imaginable way.
They also happen to be the two that I've heard more people
complain about having problems with in some aspect than any
others. These functions are sleep and elimination. Yes, we are going
to get down to it and talk about poop. But first...

Sleep

Our current mindsets, attitudes, moods, and overall abilities
to handle everyday activities absolutely depend on how much sleep
we are getting on a consistent basis. If we are consistently getting less
than seven solid (meaning as uninterrupted as possible; I know
CGMs and pumps are designed to wake us up when necessary, and
that is just part of our reality) hours of sleep per night, we are
undoubtedly suffering from that lack of sleep in various ways. We
might feel tired or depend on coffee to "pick us up" throughout the
day, have headaches, experience forgetfulness often, feel grogginess
or brain fog, experience loss of concentration or the inability to
concentrate on tasks, crankiness, or have an overall feeling of
helplessness and wanting to just give up.

These are just a few of the many symptoms of consistently
not getting enough sleep. I keep saying "consistently" because that is
a huge part of the equation. Getting eight hours one night and five
the next, then eight again, then five, and so on can absolutely still
produce any of the above-mentioned symptoms. The way we react to
everything in our lives each day, whether diabetes-related or not,
depends heavily on how well-rested our brains and bodies are.

So if you are like many of the people in the world who experience issues falling asleep, staying asleep, or getting enough hours of sleep per night, this is an area that is extremely important to focus on improving one day at a time. Nobody enjoys always feeling agitated, negative, or depressed due to a lack of adequate, quality rest. Moreover, it also affects our relationships with others, since we are always so quick to snap or are just irritable in general because we are tired.

Building muscle, losing body fat, and adapting to a new workout routine will be even more difficult for our bodies to handle if we're not sleeping 7-9 hours a night; and results will happen at a much slower pace if we are not getting at least that much sleep. I could go on and on about the unfortunate side effects of inadequate sleep, but I think I made my point. This is placed in the beginning of this section for a reason: so that I can stress, as best as possible, the incredible importance of a consistent sleep schedule in order for our bodies and brains to focus, heal, repair, and adapt every day.

Here are some helpful tips to consider when working on regulating your sleep schedule. Remember, just like anything else, these issues won't get fixed overnight (pun intended, sorry), but if we stick with them and are willing to try some different things, we can count on adding a little more time to our precious sleep schedule each week.

1. **Black-out curtains, and blacking out all of the lights in the room.** This includes alarm clocks, lights coming from cellphone chargers, and literally every speck of light. I'm talking pitch-black-can't-see-your-hand-in-front-of-your-face dark. I have black trash bags over my bedroom windows so I can enjoy the deep sleep that a pitch-black room provides. No shame in my sleep game! They sell black-out curtains at places like Walmart and K-Mart, which are very affordable.

2. **De-screening.** This is one that most of us have probably heard is helpful, but may not have been able to exert the self-control to try yet. Consciously choosing to turn off access to ALL screens 30-60 minutes before bed allows our brains to settle into a restful state. When we have the lights from a screen shining into our eyes, it signals to our brains that it's

time to be active, which is the exact opposite of what we need to settle into a restful sleep. Everything on social media will be there in the morning, and your sleep is much more important than anyone's status update!

3. **Bedtime yoga.** I know, at first, it might sound counter-productive to do anything physical before going to bed, but gentle stretching can release relaxing hormones into our systems that allow us to more easily calm down, both physically and mentally. There are countless bedtime yoga routines on *YouTube* to choose from. Doing this before bed also allows us to get out of our heads and slow down the chatter. Many of the bedtime yoga routines are designed to actually be done in bed. I realize this will require some use of a screen at first, but eventually, you will learn the stretches and can just listen to the prompts instead of staring at the screen the whole time.

4. **Meditation.** Other than the black-out curtains, this is my favorite helper, and one that I've found to be incredibly effective in helping to stop the seemingly inevitable mind-racing that pops up as soon as I lie down. Again, there are a multitude of guided meditations for sleep on *YouTube*; it's just a matter of finding one that you enjoy. I use an app on my phone called "The Oprah & Deepak 21-Day Meditation Experience." I like these because they are short (20 minutes) and meaningful, and truly allow my brain to focus on drifting off, rather than on the million things that I need to get done in my life!

5. **Sleep-inducing background noise.** I know that the word "noise" in itself might sound like something that wouldn't help us sleep, but depending on the type of noise, it can be super helpful. I personally turn on the sound of a fireplace after I finish with my meditation, through an app called "Sleep Pillow," and there are many other sleep-noise apps available. Some of us might like the sound of the ocean, while others might prefer the sound of rain, and some of us might not like any sounds at all—we are all different! Once you find what you like, it can make a huge difference in your ability to fall and stay asleep.

6. **Not having a full stomach.** Trying to fall asleep with a stomach full of food can definitely make things more difficult. Digestion is a process that will always come first in the human body. If there is food to be digested, the body will get to work on digesting it, instead of focusing on falling asleep. If you feel hungry before bed, I recommend having a small portion of something that is very quickly digested, like fruits or vegetables. Aim to eat dinner, at the very least, 2-3 hours before going to bed to get as restful a night's sleep as possible.

Elimination

The other crucial process that our bodies should be going through every day (and ideally, more than once per day) is elimination, or bowel movements, or pooping. This is one of the first things I ask new clients when getting started on any program where the goal is to create sustainable healthy habits. We can eat super healthy, exercise, and sleep really well, but if we are not pooping every day, our bodies will be in a constant state of toxicity, regardless of our other amazing efforts to improve our health. I can't tell you how many people I have encountered over the years who are not only not going every day, but are going less than three times per week. This is a very serious problem that must be addressed right away. Here are my top suggestions for getting things moving on a…regular basis:

1. **Choose to be properly hydrated all of the time.** I realize that at this point, I might sound like a broken record, but drinking a minimum of half our bodyweight in ounces of water per day can be the only thing missing from being on a regular elimination schedule. Three-quarters of an average, healthy poop is made up of water. When constipated, waste materials stay in the large intestine longer, and more water is removed, causing the feces to become hard and difficult to pass. So drink up!

2. **Eat more fiber.** It becomes easier to get enough fiber in our diets once we begin focusing on a whole-foods, nutrient-dense way of eating. Lots of vegetables, fruits, beans, nuts,

and seeds will do the trick. Some of the higher fiber items are avocados, peas, leafy greens, squash, sweet potatoes, pears, berries, chia seeds, flax seeds, apples, oranges, prunes, beans, and quinoa. These are just a few of the endless options for filling up our diets with fiber-rich foods. I recommend aiming for 30-40 grams of fiber per day.

3. **Exercise.** Seems simple enough, I know. But sometimes all it takes to get things moving, is, well, to get moving!

4. **Supplements.** I highly recommend trying all of the above options first before adding supplements, but if you've been trying consistently for over a week, using the first three options and are not seeing any results, adding a fiber supplement could do the trick. Some options I recommend are Garden of Life RAW Organic Fiber, Organic Triple Fiber by Renew Life, or Optimum Nutrition Fitness Fiber, all of which can be found on *Amazon* and other online retailers. Please be sure to stay well hydrated when taking any fiber supplements!

17

MINDFULNESS

"If you change the way you look at things, the things you look at change."
-Wayne Dyer

"Mindfulness" is a term that is (thankfully) being used more and more as the world and the humans who inhabit it grow more conscious as a whole. But what exactly does that mean, and how can we easily apply mindfulness to our day-to-day lives in order to support a healthy mind and body? My favorite definition of mindfulness that is the result of simply typing "mindfulness define" into the *Google* search bar is "a mental state achieved by focusing one's awareness on the present moment, while calmly acknowledging and accepting one's feelings, thoughts, and bodily sensations."

The act of being mindful includes aspects of all the other pillars, and gives us a term to describe putting them all together in order to create that sustainable lifestyle we desire. We must be mindful of our mindsets, nutrition, exercise, support systems, and bodily functions. Mindfulness is the foundation upon which all the other pillars can grow and flourish. Ultimately, we must be aware of the choices we are making in all those areas, and be willing to calmly and objectively acknowledge and accept our feelings, no matter what they may be moment-to-moment, without judgment.

I think, especially for my own transformation, the most challenging aspect of being mindful, and the most important aspect overall, is the ability to acknowledge what is happening with ourselves moment-to-moment *without judgment*. That is what I mean by being objective; and I must say, it takes time and practice to intentionally make this a part of who we are. And in order to be objective regarding our own thoughts, feelings, and bodily sensations, **we must first and foremost love ourselves, and accept and embrace who we are right now, where we have been, and the journey we choose to be on.**

It is virtually impossible to make positive, lasting changes in our lives if we are continually judging ourselves, and even worse, berating ourselves for the things that don't end up the way we expect them to. **Consciously practicing self-love is the most crucial element in making any sustainable changes to our habits, and is the foundation of all mindful acts.**

We must truly love ourselves; consistently give ourselves credit for all we have accomplished, big and small; and celebrate every single win, no matter how insignificant we might perceive it to be. No achievement is too small to be celebrated. If we don't love who we are and feel pride in our character as a human being, we will never fully commit to change because we won't truly feel deserving of the happiness that comes along with achieving our goals. And if we don't feel we are deserving of happiness and all of the joys that life has to offer, then no amount of effort or motivation will ever be sustained for very long.

Most people think that changing the state of our health starts with nutrition or fitness, and although these aspects are vitally important, the efforts we put into shaping our diets and exercise habits will be fleeting if we don't think we deserve the rewards that come along with them. I know this because I went through this same experience, time and time again. I started a new diet or exercise routine, and even though I began seeing some results, I eventually gave up and went back to my default settings.

I didn't know it at the time, but I now know that my giving up was due to the fact I was still holding on to the belief that I was cursed; that diabetes, the death of my father, the death of my sister, and all the other things that I experienced were forms of punishment, and that I deserved to be punished for some reason. I believed that I deserved misery and suffering, not happiness and fulfillment. Now I know that isn't true. Now I know that the truth is that bad things happen to good people all the time, and that our circumstances are not a measure of our self-worth.

The truth is that I am a good person who believes strongly in treating others the way I want to be treated, and I deserve to be happy and to experience all of the joys that life has to offer. The truth is that I deserve to feel loved, to give and receive love, and not only am I enough, but I am more than enough. And so are you. I don't care who is reading this right now, YOU are enough, and YOU deserve to feel love—to give and receive it. And the most important person to whom we all deserve to give and receive love is ourselves.

Once I was able to see how much harm I was doing to myself, completely blindly and unintentionally, emotional walls began crashing down around me, and my life was never the same again. I love me, and you must love you. And practicing mindfulness is the key to unlocking that love bit by bit, no matter how deeply we have hidden it away or how strong or large the walls we have built around it are.

One of the first things that comes to mind when thinking about acknowledging feelings without judgment are the numbers that show up on our meter or CGM screens each time we check our blood sugars. The amount of time and energy I used to spend on feeling horrible about myself, judging myself, and racking my brain for answers as to why my blood sugars weren't in range is staggering, and I know I am not the only person who has gone through this over and over again. This was a major part of my self-loathing cycle of feeling worthless and not enough and undeserving of all the joys life had to offer, all throughout my teenage years and into my 20s.

My high blood sugars meant that I was a terrible person, that I was stupid and helpless to get things right. High A1cs were even worse. Now, not only did I judge myself, but the doctors could judge me too, making my self-deprecation even more intense. The truth is that the readings on our meters are not a measure of our character, nor are they a representation of who we are as a person. High readings do not make us villains. A blood sugar reading is just that— a reading, a data point, a piece of information that allows us to make more informed and intelligent decisions about what happens next. We are lucky to have the tools and technology that allow us to make these informed decisions. And the ability to use these tools and make these decisions are in itself is a big part of what makes us superheroes.

Every single one of us living with diabetes is absolutely, positively a superhero. This superhero status, without a doubt, also includes all the moms, dads, and caretakers of children with diabetes as well. That is what a Diabetes Dominator is to me—a superhero persona that I had to create so that I could live into it, and live up to it, because I finally realized that I deserved it. The efforts and thought-cycles we must put forth day-in and day-out to live with diabetes are profound.

The fact that we must make hundreds of minute-to-minute decisions every single day just to keep ourselves alive is incredible. Every time we eat, every time we exercise, every time we sleep, every time we drive, every time we feel a bit off, a data point must be obtained and a decision must be made. The decisions that go along with taking insulin, which is the thing we need to keep ourselves alive, but also the thing that, with the wrong calculation, could kill us.

Having diabetes gives us a level of power over our health that most people will never know; and with great power comes great responsibility. I don't know of any other disease or condition that requires that amount of forethought, personal decision-making skills, and manual input on such a constant basis. We are all awesome, amazing, and impressive, and we need to embrace that. We walk a tightrope of unpredictable variables 24/7/365, and we are all superheroes whether we choose to accept it or not.

Once we are able to adopt the mentality of blood sugars, A1cs, and numbers on the scale as simple data points, bits of information that allow us to make more intelligent decisions moving forward, we begin to enter into the realm of mindfulness. Those data points are not helpful if we spend all our time judging them and allowing them to define who we believe we are as human beings, and what we do and don't deserve. But they are extremely helpful when we are able to acknowledge them without judgement in each present moment and allow them to guide our decisions about how to best proceed.

So how do we begin to bring mindfulness practices into our lives? The following are a few of the ways to integrate being more mindful into our daily habits and routines.

Practice Presence

The best time to start any new, healthy endeavor is always now, and the best place to start is always in the present moment, by becoming aware of our level of presence. What I mean by that is by being fully present in each moment of our lives, paying full attention to each encounter we have, to each experience we go through. In today's increasingly digital world, so many of us have become so wrapped up in the screens that are constantly available to us that it has unfortunately become "normal" to be texting or scrolling through social media while we are having a conversation with another person. This is very disturbing, very disrespectful, and a state of being where mindfulness cannot exist.

Our presence is, quite literally, a present—a present that we can all choose to give, both to ourselves and to others, and that has become a rare commodity, making it even more valuable. When we are looking at a screen while interacting with another person (now, of course, I'm not referring to bolusing or checking our blood sugars), we are subconsciously telling both the other person and ourselves that they are not deserving of our full attention. Further, when someone is doing that to us and we accept it as normal, we are defaulting to not being deserving of someone's full attention.

I call it "digital disrespect" (I should probably trademark that). Being mindful of other people's feelings is one of the best ways to become mindful of our own feelings. The next time you are checking out at the supermarket or any store where there is a person behind a register, set an intention to be fully present during that interaction. You will be floored to see how that person will react due to the simple fact that you are paying sole attention to them and the interaction going on at the moment.

At first, I thought this was no big deal; but now, I get great pleasure out of brightening someone else's day just by paying attention to them, and it is always a great opportunity to practice mindfulness. Try it out, I think you will be surprised at the smiles and good feelings that come of it. And imagine just how much more enriching all of our relationships and interactions would be if we did this with everyone.

Activate Awareness

Awareness and presence are very closely related. When we become present, we automatically become more aware...of everything. Aware of our feelings, aware of our thoughts, aware of our emotions, aware of our actions, and aware of the never-ending signals that our bodies are always sending us. So many of us are simply stuck on autopilot.

For example, do you have a route or exit that you always take to get home from work? Have you ever needed to go somewhere else after work instead of straight home, but instead automatically took that exit towards home because it is just the thing you are used to doing?

Another great example of ignoring our power of awareness is by texting or staring at our phones while walking down the street or through a store or anywhere else there are other people. I have seen a girl literally walk right into a telephone pole because she wasn't even slightly aware of what was going on around her. We live in a society where constant information is more abundant than ever before, and because of that, we need to consciously choose to filter how much of it to let in, and when.

We are thinking about and trying to process and compartmentalize so many things at once that it just becomes easier to go on autopilot. And sometimes, those autopilot actions create the habits that may have gotten us to a state of physical, mental, emotional, or spiritual health that are not bringing us happiness, satisfaction, or fulfillment. That is where tuning in and activating our awareness becomes an invaluable tool.

When we intentionally take the time to become aware of what is going on around us, to apply filters to the amounts and types of information we choose to consume, to listen to our bodies and become aware of the signals they are sending us, that is when the changes we are trying to make permanent finally begin to stick. Being present in each moment and actively being aware of each situation we are in make mindfulness part of our reality.

Create Clarity

Getting clear on exactly what we want is a game-changer. Being fully intentional about and focused on the specific outcomes we are aiming to achieve are key to actually knowing when we have reached success on our own terms. Defining what success means to each of us is paramount. If we don't put exact parameters, benchmarks, and milestones on our route to achieving any goal, then we won't be able to recognize when we have become successful.

We must be able to recognize success, and the only way to do that is to be crystal clear on what success means to us individually.

This means not going by someone else's definition of success (although I highly recommend talking to and/or studying or reading up on people who you feel are successful, and see what their habits and practices are). This means that YOU decide what success looks like at every step along the path so that as soon as you see it, you immediately recognize and CELEBRATE it. That is the secret to sustaining motivation.

Being motivated to get started is something we've all experienced, but keeping that motivation alive is where many of us struggle. Creating clarity on what success means, and defining very specific, realistic, and attainable benchmarks along the way will allow our motivation to continually be stoked and renewed. We need to feel successful on a regular basis in order to stay motivated to keep moving forward. Because without the celebrations of hitting milestones of success along the way to the ultimate goal, there is nothing giving us hope or the satisfaction of knowing that we are still heading in the right direction. So let's get clear on those milestones of success along the way, and be mindful to celebrate and give ourselves credit all throughout the journey.

The Mind-Body Connection

Now for a word on the mind-body connection, or psychoneuroimmunology (PNI for short). Merriam-Webster defines psychoneuroimmunology as "a branch of medicine that deals with the influence of emotional states (as stress) and nervous system activities on immune function." This is a long definition for what I like to think of much more simply as how incredibly powerful and mind-blowingly profound our mind-body connection really is. The thoughts we have, the beliefs we hold, and the language we use not only influence our emotional states, but I genuinely believe they also have a stark and real effect on our health and wellbeing.

> *"Whether you think you can, or you think you can't--you're right."*
> -Henry Ford

Now, don't get me wrong here. I'm NOT saying that we can think diabetes away or anything like that. What I am saying is that if we consistently think and feel that we are ill in any number of ways, our brains and bodies will physically react in turn. I have not only personally experienced this myself (with my bout with cancerous cells in my cervix), but have also read extensively on the subject and seen it come to fruition with many other people. And if we genuinely believe that we are not sick in any number of ways, our bodies will physically react to that as well.

The immune system and the brain "talk" to each other through signaling pathways, and this process is crucial for maintaining homeostasis. The brain and the immune system are the two major adaptive systems of the body. Again, I can't stress enough that I, in no way, aim to blame anyone or say that anyone could've prevented any illness that they have experienced or are experiencing. I am aiming to illustrate, beyond all doubt, that our thoughts become actual things, and that when we are able to become aware of and recognize this powerful connection, we can use it to our advantage.

I can't tell you how many times over the years that both my husband and I have felt a cold or flu-like symptoms coming on, and/or have been exposed to other people who were contagiously sick in any number of ways. And instead of just accepting that it was inevitable that we would get sick too, we clearly and intentionally stated repeatedly that not only were we not sick, but we would not allow those feelings to manifest any further. Add some extra water, green vegetables, and some Vitamin B and C to the mix, and I have not had the flu since I was 16 years old. And I cannot remember the last time I had a cold.

Is it because I use the incredible power of my brain to direct my immune system? I can't say for sure. But I can say for sure that my husband and I (almost) never get sick, as compared to the frequency at which I hear others report that they are suffering from any number of cold/virus symptoms, and I believe it is, in part, because we adamantly choose to use our brain powers to influence our immune systems.

PNI can be explained in another way: the placebo effect. The placebo effect is related to the perceptions and expectations of the individual. If the placebo is viewed as helpful, it can heal. If the placebo is viewed as harmful, the nocebo effect, it can cause negative effects; when, in reality, it was nothing at all, one way or the other. How many times have we heard of a long married couple where one of the partners passes away, only for the other to pass shortly thereafter, when there was no illness present in the other partner whatsoever? Clearly our mind-body connection has a strong influence on our health and wellbeing. And while it's nice that there are science and experiments to back it up, you only have to check in with yourself to see if it makes sense for you.

Now, here's the thing—maybe I'm as cuckoo as an old clock—but, and this is the real thing here, I BELIEVE with every fiber of my being that I have this iron-clad mind-body connection, and it has served me unrelentingly over the years. Through minor things like colds and flus, and major things like cancer cells in my cervix, I REFUSED to allow my brain to signal to my body that these things were happening. I made a choice to let my brain know that these things were simply not acceptable and will not be tolerated in any capacity. And my signaling pathways—my immune system and my brain, my two major adaptive systems in my body—have heard my directions loud and clear.

And at the end of the day, what we believe to be true with total certainty is our reality. So, my point is that our thoughts and our beliefs shape our realities, no matter whether or not anyone else in the world believes they are true. You have this same power. Don't accept anything as inevitable. Don't decide that since you were in a room full of sneezing kids that you are destined to catch that cold. Don't believe that just because you got some preliminary, unverified diagnosis of anything that you are destined to travel that road.

Because if you do have the power to influence your immune response, even if there is just the tiniest chance that this is all true, wouldn't you rather say "hell no" to any disease state that may or may not be in your body, than to simply sit back and succumb to whatever may be? I know I would. And I believe with all my heart that you have this power too, and I encourage you to try it out.

But the catch is, if you don't believe it will work, it probably won't; because what you believe with total certainty is your reality. Back it up with some real faith and put it to the test. I think you will be pleasantly surprised at the results. If not, file me under the cuckoo clock category on this one and move on!

Avoid "I Already Know That" Syndrome

What does that mean? I believe that each and every one of us, at some point in our lives, has experienced what I call "I Already Know That Syndrome". It is a killer of mindfulness, and also creates a closed-mind to what can often be very important topics. It might flare up when we are listening to our doctor talk about how important regular exercise is to our blood sugar management, or when we hear our CDE or nutritionist tell us that eating less carbs and processed foods is the best way to reach that A1c under seven that we've been chasing.

It inevitably pops into our heads…YES, I already KNOW that! But that's the thing…there is a massive difference between knowing and doing, between awareness and application. That is one of the reasons I made it a priority to strike that term from my vocabulary. Because unless I am practicing that thing daily and it is a part of who I am, I don't really know it.

When we say "I already know that," we are telling our brains that it is okay for us to dismiss whatever it is that is being said, and that it's not important information. We are also giving ourselves permission to tune-out and not actively and mindfully listen to what is being said. And I've found over the years that we do this most often when what is being said is something we know we should be doing for the benefit of our own wellbeing, but are not doing consistently or at all.

"I already know that" is the perfect excuse for automatically downgrading the importance of the information we are hearing, no matter how incredibly important it might actually be. I had to practice eradicating that term from my life. The way I did that (and still do it, because it absolutely still happens to this day) is to catch myself in the act. If I'm listening to a presentation at a conference, for example, and the speaker says something that triggers the "I already know that" syndrome, I immediately catch myself and ask, "Do you really already know that?" Occasionally the answer is "yes," but only if it is something that I think is valuable that I've already fully integrated into my life.

If it is information that I find to be valuable but do not currently practice, but know that if I did practice would benefit my overall wellbeing, I tell myself explicitly that I don't already know that and to tune-in and pay closer attention. Next time you find yourself experiencing "I Already Know That" syndrome, pause and honestly assess if you really do already know that and have fully integrated it into your life, or if your brain is simply looking for a reason to tune it out because you don't want to mindfully experience any negative feelings surrounding the fact that you are not currently doing what is being said, even though you know it would add value to your life.

Tips for Practicing Presence, Activating Awareness, and Creating Clarity

It's important to have a high-level overview of what these things actually mean in respect to our lives, but even more important is to immerse ourselves in the daily practices that allow us to integrate them into our being. Here are my top four daily practices that have allowed me to go from zero to mindful in just minutes a day. Start with one of these practices at a time (don't overload yourself all at once) and add a new one each week or month, depending on how soon you feel ready. Simply adding one of these practices to our lives on a daily basis will help to make mindfulness our new default setting!

Morning Routine

As people living with diabetes, we know that the more predictable our routines are, the more predictable our diabetes management practices can be. When it comes to having a specific, pre-planned morning routine, not only will it take any guesswork out of what we are going to do in the morning, which helps us avoid chaos and confusion, but it will also help us get out of bed with more purpose. Having a morning routine allows us to practice not only mindfulness, but also self-love, by choosing to dedicate time to ourselves with the direct intention of nurturing our health and well-being—because we embrace that we deserve it.

Just like we all need to create our own individual nutritional lifestyles that work best for us, each of us needs to create a morning routine that best fits into our lives. Some of us might have a ten-minute morning routine, and some of us might have one that lasts an hour or more. It's not the amount of time that is most important; it is the full commitment to blocking out that time for ourselves no matter what, and not letting anything get in the way. Our morning routine time is sacred.

That means NO phone calls, NO checking e-mails, NO looking at social media. It means not letting anyone else's priorities or agenda come before ours, at least during that sacred time. A morning routine can consist of many things; there are no right or wrong answers (unless we are submitting to someone else's agenda and not putting nurturing ourselves as our top priority), and we must choose what we want ours to consist of.

Making the time to give ourselves this gift is a necessity. No matter what time I have to get up or for what reason, I make sure I factor in the time it will take for me to get through these few practices so I can set myself up for success, and feel confident that I will be prepared to handle anything the rest of the day brings. I think you will be surprised at how much just 10-15 minutes dedicated to yourself in the morning will begin to positively shape the outcomes of the rest of the day.

Here are some examples of things that are part of my morning routine:

1. **Hydration:** Immediately upon opening my eyes (after checking my CGM and pump, making any correction boluses if necessary, and increasing my basal rates by 60-80% for the first 1-2 hours of the day…dawn phenomenon!), I reach over to my nightstand, grab my water bottle, and proceed to drink 16 ounces or more of water. Our bodies need hydration first thing in the morning to get things going, especially since we've just gone (hopefully) eight hours without drinking any water. This all takes under three minutes.

2. **Meditation:** Another part of my morning routine is ten minutes of meditation that I usually do while still in bed. This allows me to calm my mind and get set-up to win the day, instead of just hitting the ground running and not allowing my mind any time to calmly adjust from sleeping to being fully awake. It also gives me time to set intentions for what outcomes I want to achieve by the time I get back into bed later that night.

3. **Gratitude Journal:** This is a simple (yet incredibly profound) notebook that sits on the nightstand by my bed. When I start

the day out by writing down one or two things for which I am truly grateful and why, it sets up my state of mind to more easily feel happy for what I am blessed to have in my life. It also serves as an intensely powerful tool to use when I am feeling down, as I can go pick up my journal and read through it to reflect on all of the things I've written down over time, anytime I need a reminder of all the things I have to be grateful for. I also repeat this step before going to bed because it is just that awesome and makes such a huge difference in my quality of life. This generally takes about five minutes.

4. **Physical Movement:** I'm not big into heavy morning workouts (but if you are, more power to you, and that is an excellent part of a morning routine and a way to dedicate time and energy to your wellbeing) so depending on the day, I might do ten minutes of gentle yoga stretching, ten minutes of light bouncing on my rebounder, or sometimes a bit of cardio by going to the park for a walk/jog, or getting on the elliptical. This could take anywhere from ten minutes to an hour, depending on what the day looks like and how I'm feeling.

5. **Daily Planner:** After I've hydrated, meditated, practiced gratitude, and moved my body, it's time to sit down and plan out my day. And now that I've taken the time to nourish my mind and body and show myself the love I deserve, my mind and body are more willing to carry me through the day, no matter how intense or jam-packed it might be.

Realistically speaking, as long as it's not a day where I go do cardio, I can get all five items in my morning routine completed in less than 40 minutes. After I began consistently integrating these practices into my life (and I've had countless clients tell me the same), my anxiety and stress levels were greatly reduced throughout all aspects of life, especially regarding my diabetes management. Starting with just one of the above mentioned practices can really make a huge difference in all aspects of our lives. Having a morning routine sets up a solid foundation from which to build on for the rest of the day—a foundation of practiced mindfulness and self-love whose benefits are truly never-ending.

A Note on Dawn Phenomenon

Whether one has diabetes or not, all humans experience what those of us living with diabetes become acutely aware of because of its effects, and refer to as "dawn phenomenon." In very simple terms, when we wake from a restful state after sleeping all night, our bodies experience a surge of hormonal activities that are related to our natural circadian rhythms, getting our bodies ready to get up and face the day. For those of us with diabetes, whose pancreases are unable to produce insulin to battle the rising blood sugars that often accompany dawn phenomenon, we can be left with higher blood sugars in the morning for what seems like no reason.

That is why I personally, through experimentation, have found that I need to set a temporary basal rate on my pump the second I open my eyes of about 60-80% for about 1-2 hours most days. If this is something you are experiencing, I recommend experimenting to see what works best for you to offset the morning highs. If you are using a pump, it could mean trying a temporary basal rate, first for one hour, then extending longer if you need it.

If you are manually injecting, it could mean taking a half-unit, whole unit, or more upon waking up, on top of any correction factor you are already giving if needed. Again, what will work for each person can vary wildly, and must be based on any number of factors. These can include what your blood sugars are when you wake up, and what your plans are for the immediate future, such as when and what you are going to eat, are you going to go exercise, etc. This is just another part of our individual science experiment that we must figure out to the best of our abilities. And some of us might not notice its effects at all!

PART FOUR - TAKE ACTION

YOUR FIRST 30 DAYS OF ADOPTING DIABETES DOMINATOR MINDSETS AND HABITS - REPETITION IS THE MOTHER OF SKILL

18

PREPARATION

"Success isn't an overnight thing. It's when every day you get a little better than the day before. It all adds up."
-Dwayne "The Rock" Johnson

This is the "take action" section, so as you may have guessed, it's time to take the lessons from above six pillars and make a plan on how to put them into action. This is the time to get those phones out and get ready to set alerts and reminders, and to schedule the things you will choose to focus on first in order to set a solid foundation to build on and support your sustainable healthy lifestyle. Because the truth is, the basics are the foundation, and simplicity is key. Taking directed measures NOT to overcomplicate things when first getting started is crucial to allowing ourselves to hit those milestones and sustain our motivation along the way to reaching our goals. It is too easy to lose sight of the basics and to overcomplicate things from the start.

We will go through each pillar and lay out the specific actions that need to be taken in order to adopt new healthy habits, so there is no confusion or guesswork regarding what needs to get done. It is up to you to choose where to start. Using the Wheel of Total Health in Part 2 of this book is a great indicator of where you will be best served to focus the most attention first.

Then slowly build upon each pillar until you are well on your way to where you want to be. We must always keep in mind that repetition is the mother of skill. We can't get good at anything or develop solid habits of any kind without repeating them over and over again until they are truly a part of our learned skillset.

In order to maximize the efforts we put forth over the next 30 days, it is crucial to keep in mind that our mentality, attitude, and ability to stay strong in the face of what are sure to be times when things don't go according to plan are going to be the deciding factors on whether or not these new habits we are trying to form actually stick for the long-run. Our willingness to admit when we are wrong and make mistakes; to recognize when we are defaulting to old beliefs that aren't serving us; and more importantly, to not let those mistakes snowball into additional poor choices are all things we need to remain aware of. Our ability to acknowledge, without judgment, that we may make choices that aren't in our plans, and to get back on the original plans right away is paramount.

We must also embrace that our attitudes and willingness to practice mindfulness, specifically regarding how we react to external stimuli that we cannot control (friends, family, co-workers, the weather, the outcome of sporting events, and all things we cannot control but too often dictate how we feel), will always determine the outcome of every single thing that ever happens to us. If it is raining outside and we decide that means we get to slack off because the weather isn't ideal, or if one of our co-workers snaps at us or doesn't do their job the way we think they should, and we are angry and in a bad mood for the rest of the day, these are examples of letting external stimuli determine our realities.

We cannot allow things that are out of our control determine the realities of our day-to-day lives. I believe with all of my being that every day above ground is a good day. We must focus on the things we can control, and I believe the only things each of us really can control are our choices.

> *"It is in our moments of decision that our destinies are shaped."*
> -Tony Robbins

Proactive Versus Reactive

When it comes to taking action, the most important job we all have is to be PROACTIVE instead of REACTIVE. For example, instead of waiting for our blood sugar to be 200 before correcting, we choose to set reminder alarms on our phones to go off each hour, so we are checking our blood sugars too often for them get that high without our knowing as often as possible. This means that if we wear a CGM, we choose to set our high alert lines lower than 200 which is the factory setting (mine is at 130 after years of slowly bringing it down a little at a time; bringing it down lower too fast can be stressful) so we can become aware of rising blood sugars and have the ability to make informed decisions about correcting before it gets too far out of range. Just because the factory setting is at 200 does not mean that is where we need to keep it; ultimately, that is up to each of us to decide.

Being proactive instead of reactive means taking the time to plan our meals out each week, and shop for and prepare some meals and healthy snacks so when it's time to eat, we already know what we have available to us, instead of standing in front of the refrigerator wondering what we should have. Being proactive versus reactive means taking the time to stash glucose tabs, glucose gel, juice boxes, or any combination of the three EVERYWHERE so when lows hit us like a ton of bricks, as they are known to do, we have a way to treat it at our fingertips at all times.

Stash them in the kitchen, living room, bedroom, car, basement, your purse/backpack/diabetes supply pack, at your best friend's house. Literally everywhere you spend time, there must be low blood sugar treatment options; but most importantly, always keep them on your person for those inevitable times we are out shopping and get what Melissa Lee, Interim Executive Director of the Diabetes Hands Foundation, so accurately coins as "shop-o-glycemia." It is nobody's responsibility but our own to be prepared for these inevitable occurrences, to be proactive versus reactive.

This can be applied to every single one of the six pillars, and is the key to lasting success in all aspects of a sustainable healthy lifestyle. Being a Diabetes Dominator means that we are willing to put our health first and foremost over all else so we can give the very best of who we are to all areas and relationships in our lives, instead of the always reactive, often frazzled and overwhelmed version of ourselves.

What all of this means is that we will have to do new things, things we aren't used to doing, things that make us uncomfortable, and we will have to do them repeatedly until they no longer make us feel that way. That is how we expand our comfort zones. Your current comfort zone is likely what led you to where you are now—reading this book and looking to change your health habits and your relationship with diabetes because you are not happy with where they are right now. All growth and progress is made outside of our comfort zones, so it serves us all to be willing to feel uncomfortable. They aren't called growing pains for nothing!

19

TAKE ACTION: MINDSET

"An optimist sees an opportunity in every calamity; a pessimist sees a calamity in every opportunity."
-Winston Churchill

1. **Gratitude Stacking.** The easiest way to change our attitudes and our overall psychology is to choose to get grateful. What I mean by this is to specifically take time out each day to be still, sit quietly, reflect, and breathe deeply, even if it's only for 3-5 minutes. Sit quietly with your hand over your heart and your eyes closed, and concentrate on any and all of the reasons you have to be grateful—the more things you can stack up, the better (this is the same Gratitude Stacking Action Item from the Mindset section). It might be for the love of your family and friends, for your job, for your health, for your strength, for being a diabetes superhero, for your pets, for nature, for Earth, or for anything you have ever accomplished in your life, no matter how big or small it might seem.

   We can be grateful for winning an award, graduating from school, for the water that runs out of your faucets, for the heat that comes out of your vents, for the roof over your head. Gratitude is an extremely powerful feeling that fuels positivity. Gratitude and anger cannot exist together, nor gratitude and fear. Gratitude is more powerful than anger and fear combined, so it is a wise choice to use it as a weapon against both of those negative emotions any time they arise. It is a tool that is free to all human beings, and one that is at our disposal at all times at the snap of a finger. The more often we allow ourselves to get grateful, the easier it will be to snap into that state of mind in the future at any given moment, no matter what may be going on around us. Choose to be grateful on a consistent basis and watch your life and the ways in which you perceive things inevitably change for the better.

2. **Ask Productive Questions.** In order to begin conditioning our minds to more automatically use language that will serve us on making progress and staying on track with things like lowering our blood sugars, reducing our medications, body fat percentage, and fears, we must be willing to ask ourselves the following questions every day, and not put the notebook down until we come up with at least two answers for each of them. Keep a notebook by your bedside (this can be separate from your gratitude journal, or get one of those two-section notebooks, and keep all of this awesomeness in one notebook). Keeping it there makes us look at it as soon as we wake up and before we go to bed, and the more visual reminders we have to keep ourselves on track, the better. This simple and meaningful exercise will set your mind up for success every single time.

Morning Questions:

1. What am I grateful for in my life right now? What about that makes me grateful? How does that make me feel?

2. What am I proud of in my life right now? What about that makes me proud? How does that make me feel?

3. What am I focused on that will enrich my life and the lives of others right now? What about that keeps me focused? How does that make me feel?

Evening Questions:

1. What have I given today, either to myself or to others?

2. What did I learn today?

3. How has today added to the quality of my life or to the quality of life of others?

3. **Make a Vision Board.** Not only can making a vision board be incredibly helpful in keeping us on track by giving us a constant visual reference of what it is that we are trying to achieve, but it can also be a very therapeutic and uplifting exercise for our creative expression that we can do as many times as we want. When constructing a vision board, the only limit is your imagination. Use colorful markers, print out photos from the internet, or just write your goals in big lettering so you are reminded on a consistent basis of what it is you truly want out of both your health and your life.

Another of my favorite quotes that really applies when it comes to making vision boards is from Ellen Johnson Sirleaf: "If your dreams do not scare you, they are not big enough." There is no dream too big or outlandish for our vision boards, ESPECIALLY if you have no idea how it will ever happen; that is all the more reason to put that vision up there and out into the universe. It is not the how that matters, it is the WHY. The WHY will guide us in the direction of the how, bit by bit. The more we see things, the more we focus on them, and the more space they occupy in our brains.

Like I've said before, where our focus goes, our energy flows. Make a vision board for your bedroom, for your living room, for any room you spend a lot of time in. My vision board is hanging on the wall directly behind my front door, so it is the first thing I see as soon as I walk into the house, and every time I go from the living room to upstairs, and vice versa. It is also directly visible from my work station. So I see it all day, every day, and I am constantly reminded of the goals I have set for myself, which is especially helpful on those days we all have when it is hard to pull ourselves together and get moving. Having a vision board is like having a pleasant kick in the butt when our motivation is low. And I can't tell you how gratifying it is to put little checkmarks or smiley faces next to the goals/pictures when they come true. The feelings of fulfillment and pride are immense and immeasurable.

4. **Manage What You Measure.** Only weigh yourself once a week, on the same day, at the same time, and wearing the same thing, preferably naked. Those of us living with diabetes have enough numbers and data points to consider every day. How much we weigh is a data point that is not important to concern our brains with on a daily basis, and one that can unnecessarily cause many of us to feel bad about ourselves if we let it. So many people get caught up in staring at the number on the scale every single day, and don't realize that it is not even close to being the best way to track progress.

   A much better and more reliable way to gauge how our bodies have changed week to week or month to month is choosing a piece of clothing that does not fit us right now, and trying it on once a week or once a month to see how much closer to fitting it is. Another reliable way to track progress regarding how our bodies are reshaping and restructuring is by taking pictures once a month, again making sure to wear the same thing each time. The best way to track progress is by taking our measurements once a month and counting inches lost, versus just relying on the scale.

5. **Can the Criticism.** Do not beat yourself up or insult yourself. Trust me, I know that's easier said than done, and we are all our own worst critics, myself included. However, in order to make permanent changes and make new habits stick for good, we all need to be our own number-one fan, cheerleader, and support system. If we begin to stray from our healthy choices, we must not default to insulting ourselves. Do not falsely convince yourself that you've ruined all effort put in thus far, and that you might as well just veer off track for the rest of the day/week/month. Don't choose self-sabotage— aka, take the easy way out.

Recognize your mistake, learn from it, and move on. Catch yourself in the act of beating yourself up, and stop doing it. Revert immediately to gratitude stacking, changing your physiology (get up and move your body), or reach out for support. The more time we spend focusing on negative things, the more negativity will manifest itself in our lives. It is also very important to celebrate every victory we achieve, no matter how small it might seem, and never forget that there is no victory too small to celebrate. This means that every time we finish a workout, every time we eat a healthy meal, every time we drink our required ounces of water in a day, we must pat ourselves on the back and tell ourselves that we are awesome, that we deserve to feel accomplished and proud of ourselves, that we are worth the time it takes, and that we deserve to feel healthy and vibrant.

Verbally congratulate yourself. Put on your favorite song and dance around the house. As silly as it might seem, this positive reinforcement trains our brains to become addicted to all those good things we are doing, which in turn causes an incredible upward spiral. Talking to ourselves, although jokingly might sound silly, is such an important aspect of creating new habits and staying on track.

6. **Embrace your Super Powers.** As individuals, we all have our own personal power. What that ultimately means is that we have the powers of **choice and decision**. We use our power of choice every moment of every day, whether we are aware (mindful) of it or not. We choose to get out of bed or not get out of bed in the morning, to exercise or not exercise, to eat breakfast or not eat breakfast, to check our blood sugar or not check our blood sugar. Every single thing we do or don't do is a choice, and it is a scary amount of power when you really think about it.

We can choose to use our power of choice for good or for evil. We must harness our own personal power for things that will make us feel good, like eating healthy food and exercising regularly; instead of on things we know will bring us pain in the long-run, like eating processed food and staying sedentary, which leads to gaining fat, losing muscle mass, and having less energy and confidence. When we make a choice, we are ultimately making a decision.

The Latin translation of the word "decision" literally means "to cut off," meaning to cut off from any other possibilities. In other words, it means to commit fully to one choice, which is what we do when we make any choice, good or bad. We commit to running a 5k, or we commit to finishing an entire pint of Ben and Jerry's; either way, we choose, we commit, and we get it done! The willingness to understand, accept, and embrace how powerful each and every one of our choices are is crucial. Choose to become more aware of your personal power of choice, and exercise it more consistently and intentionally, instead of just going with the flow and agenda of other people's choices. This requires opening our minds. This requires not dismissing something just because it doesn't work out immediately. We must choose to reassess and retry. Simply being aware of information or ideas we didn't know before will begin to subconsciously shape our decision-making processes.

Choose these tools any time you feel like your mindset isn't on course with your goals. Just like any habit we set out to form, having the right mindset must be practiced, so don't let your attitude get too far out of control before you check yourself, verbally or otherwise. Sit quietly and get grateful. Spend a few minutes working on your daily questions. Get up and do 30 jumping jacks with a huge smile on your face, even if it is fake. I guarantee that by the end of the 30 jumping jacks, you will feel a very real change in your mental state, and that's the goal. Choose to step into your power of choice, the choice to change your mindset anytime you want. Understand, accept, and embrace your power to choose and change how you feel at any given moment.

20

TAKE ACTION: NUTRITION

"A person who never made a mistake never tried anything new."
-Albert Einstein

It's time to get started in the kitchen, to take actions that are specifically directed at creating a supportive environment that will assist you in reaching your nutritional goals. The action items listed below are all very real choices we all must make, and the sooner we get them done, the better. These things are all ways to begin exercising your power of choice and taking control of one of the very few things we as human beings truly have control over: what we choose to eat and not eat. Let's get started!

1. **Kitchen/Pantry/Cabinet Cleanout.** The VERY FIRST thing that everyone needs to do in order to succeed during this first 30 days, and really for as long as you want to live in an environment that is supportive of a healthy nutritional lifestyle, is to take full stock of and clean out your kitchen. This includes all areas, such as your fridge, pantry, shelves, cabinets, and anywhere else you might be storing (or hiding, like I used to do) any unhealthy, non-nutrient-dense, non-whole, processed foods. You must adopt and follow the "out with the old, in with the new" mentality in order to truly allow yourself the ability to transform your current nutritional habits and lifestyle.

    Take all the foods you are choosing not to eat (that are unopened) to a local food bank or anywhere that accepts food donations. When we clean out our kitchen, we are not only making room for new, healthier options, but also helping ourselves feel like we have already gotten a bit lighter by relieving ourselves of the space those junky foods were taking up in our minds. Download my "Healthy & Unhealthy" pantry clean-out guide and shopping list guide as references at **diabetesdominator.com.**

2. **Make a Plan.** Now that your kitchen is clean and clear of unhealthy options, it is time to take a few minutes and plan your meals for the upcoming week. Planning ahead is the cornerstone to success. As cliché as it is, failing to plan is planning to fail. Below, I have included some suggestions for a week's worth of meals, as well as a number of healthy recipes. These are great guides to use to get started, and then you can build your ideal nutritional lifestyle from there. This is also a good time to surf the web and find other recipes that are quick and easy, so you can fill in your breakfast, lunch, dinner, and snacks for one week.

   I'm a big fan of crockpot meals, where you can just throw everything in one pot, turn it on, walk away, and come back to a delicious, healthy meal that will also yield plenty of leftovers for the rest of the week. This planning time is a time slot that MUST be scheduled into our calendars every single week. Even when we start to get the hang of it, it is still crucial to take the time to sit down and make a plan. It's too easy to think that we have a handle on it because we've done it for a few weeks in a row, and then skip that planning session and watch the next week fall apart at the seams.

3. **Make a List and Go Shopping.** A very important action that we ALWAYS need to take to keep ourselves focused and on-track at the supermarket is to make a list beforehand of what we need, and make a personal rule NOT to deviate from that list. Go in, cross off the list items, and get out. All of us know that the supermarket can be an evil place if we are not prepared before we walk in.

   Based on the meals and recipes you chose in step two for your meals for the upcoming week, make a shopping list specifically to support your ability to prepare those meals and snacks. ONLY after your list is complete, head to the local farmer's market, supermarket, or wherever you go to buy food, so you can consciously and intentionally re-stock your kitchen with the ingredients you need to succeed!

4. **Prep and Cook.** Now that you have a clean and clear kitchen, a written plan for your meals for the upcoming week, and you have gone shopping for all the ingredients you need, it's time to get cooking. Setting aside and committing a couple of hours each week to preparing the foods you plan on eating during the upcoming week is a non-negotiable step in sustaining healthy eating habits.

   There is also the option of choosing a home-delivery meal service. These have become more and more available nowadays, and many deliver already-prepared, healthy meals right to your door. I have never used these options myself, but have heard good things. I imagine having the food delivered is more costly than doing it yourself, but if that's a viable option for you, and the company is health-centered, I say go for it.

5. **Portion Control.** Once your meals and snacks are all ready to go, the final step is dividing them up into individual containers that are ready for you to grab-and-go all throughout the week. I can't tell you the amount of stress relief having this done ahead of time can provide. It frees up our minds and our focus in such a major way. So many of us go through the same exact thought processes, day after day, of "what am I going to have for breakfast/lunch/dinner/snacks?"

   Once your meals are prepped and portioned, the freedom it will allow your mind can be overwhelming at first. No more thought-cycles have to be spent on what you are going to eat, until the week is over and you plan for the next week. That level of freedom is invaluable, and one that many of us never experience. Give yourself the gift of a clearer mind and a healthier body, because you deserve it.

6. **MyFitnessPal.com (MFP).** If you haven't already done so, set up your personal account on www.myfitnesspal.com and download the app to your phone. This is one of the most important tools we need to succeed from here on out. See the "Nutrition" section for step-by-step details regarding how to personalize your MFP account.

7. **Low Blood Sugar Preparedness.** Part of creating a healthy nutritional lifestyle that will serve us for the rest of our lives is to choose to embrace that experiencing low blood sugars (hypoglycemia) is a medical issue and needs to be treated as such. It is not a time designated for treats like candy, cookies, etc. It is a serious issue that, in order to maintain a healthy mindset around nutrition, needs to be taken care of with glucose tabs, glucose gel, or 100% juice boxes. One of my biggest downfalls when I was in a very unhealthy mindset and nutritional lifestyle was that I saw having a low blood sugar as a chance to eat whatever I wanted—a sort of free-time to eat whatever unhealthy items I could get my hands on.

When we get into this habit, it unconsciously trains our brains to look forward to low blood sugars because we designate it as a time to have a "treat" without the usual guilt we might feel if we ate those things while our blood sugar wasn't low. This is a dangerous habit and one that I know many people with diabetes have. We must consciously choose to treat hypoglycemia with something that we wouldn't want to consume if our blood sugars weren't low, such as the glucose tabs, gel, or juice boxes. Having low blood sugars aren't an excuse to reward ourselves.

Another huge advantage to this is that the less we treat ourselves with junky foods, the more in control we are of the dreaded over-treating of the lows. If we have a treatment method that is clearly marked and always readily available to us (glucose tabs = 4 grams of carbs per tab, glucose gel = 15 grams of carbs per packet, juice box = anywhere from 15-25 grams of carbs per box), we are MUCH more in control of the amount of carbs we consume, therefore making it much less likely that we will eat 50-100 grams of carbs to treat a low that really only requires 15-30 grams of carbs.

Being prepared by putting these things on our shopping lists, setting reminders in our phones to restock weekly, and making sure these treatment options are ALWAYS available to us everywhere (kitchen, bedroom, living room, basement, car, purse, backpack, friend's house, etc.) makes it an automatic reaction to reach for these things when lows hit. This takes away the need to stand shaking, staring at the kitchen, totally confused about what to eat, and then eating everything in sight. An ounce of preparation can save us countless pounds of over-treating lows, as well as keep us off of the dreaded blood sugar roller-coaster, more often than not. Again, this is yet another choice that we all have. It is up to each of us to make sure we are prepared for lows; it's nobody's responsibility but our own, even though it downright sucks.

Like I've mentioned previously, each person will need to experiment to find what foods and meals work best for each of our bodies and lifestyles. The "Healthy & Unhealthy" food lists, as well as the following meal plan suggestions are only guidelines to help you get started. They are not a bible that must be followed to the T, or else you get struck down by the blood sugar gods! They are meant to serve as a foundation from which you can build your own healthy lifestyle, because only you can decide what truly works best for your body.

For the first 30 days of creating new habits, I highly recommend eliminating as many as possible (preferably all) of the foods from the "Unhealthy" food list so your body has some time to cleanse and detoxify. During any periods of detoxification and changing of nutritional habits, it is normal and expected to experience some level of discomfort. Anything from cold-like symptoms, to low energy, to irritability, to skin rash, to anything else in between are possible discomforts. This is your body's way of pushing the toxins to the surface and OUT of your cells. Like I mentioned before, we have to be willing to be uncomfortable during times of change.

Here are a few basic guidelines to follow to create some structure when getting started:

1. Eat breakfast.
2. Aim to not let more than four hours go by without eating something.
3. Pre-bolus for meals in order to best mitigate post-meal blood sugar spikes. Use MFP or a website like **www.calorieking.com** to determine how many carbs are in your upcoming meal.
4. Eat the majority of your daily calories during breakfast, lunch, and day-time snacks so that your body has a chance to use that fuel during the day. Have a smaller dinner so your body is not bogged down by digestion and fluctuating blood sugar levels when you are trying to get to sleep.
5. If you want a snack after dinner, choose something that is higher in protein and fat and lower in carbohydrates, such as raw cashews or almonds; a can of tuna, salmon, or sardines; or, my favorite, a sliced avocado with lime juice, salt, pepper, and chopped-up mint or basil.

ACTION ITEM: I prepared a 5 day sample meal plan for you! View and print (or copy) the meal plan to get a good idea of some nutrient dense and delicious meals for your week. Get your meal plan here: diabetesdominator.com/mealplan

I can't stress enough that these meal suggestions are simply foundations for you to build your own nutritional lifestyle from. If you see a recipe that you like that has something in it that you don't like, MODIFY IT TO YOUR LIKING! There is a reason I'm only giving you five days' worth of suggestions. It is because it is crucial to focus on learning, understanding, and implementing foods that are healthy, fit into your lifestyle, and make you happy, ON YOUR OWN.

This transformation is as much about your becoming empowered and confident about building your own meals from now on, as it is about learning to eat healthy consistently. Unless you have a personal chef, YOU are the only one who is responsible for what you eat, so take these next 30 days as a crash-course learning experience, pay attention, take notes, look up and use recipes, and build your confidence for making healthy decisions for yourself from now on!

Some Recommended Products:

I get most of these products at my local supermarket, or at Whole Foods or Trader Joe's. Whatever I can't find there, I order from *Amazon* and other online retailers.

*Nutiva chia seeds
*Optimum Nutrition Fitness Fiber
*Nature's Promise organic almond butter and peanut butter
*Crazy Richard's peanut butter
*Wild Friends nut and seed butters
*Native Forest organic unsweetened coconut milk (canned)
*Eden organic pumpkin seeds
*Dang toasted coconut chips lightly salted (no sugar added)
*Go Raw bars
*Nutritional yeast flakes
*Coconut Secret coconut aminos (in place of soy sauce)
*Brad's raw kale chips
*Lily's chocolate bars
*Celtic sea salt or real salt
*Amy's low sodium refried beans
*Amy's low sodium split pea soup and lentil vegetable soup (note: some Amy's brand soups have added sugars/carbs, so be sure to read the label)
*Organicville tomato basil marinara sauce
*L.E. Roselli marinara sauce
*Optimum Nutrition Gold Standard whey protein powder
*MRM Veggie Elite protein powder
*Vega One and Vega Sport protein powder
*Mary's Gone Crackers brand crackers
*Mrs. Dash seasonings
*Frontier brand seasonings
*Cold-pressed olive, almond, coconut, and avocado oils

*PUR brand chewing gum
*Wild Planet sardines
*Gimme organic roasted seaweed snacks

21

TAKE ACTION: EXERCISE

"The greatest glory in living lies not in never falling, but in rising every time we fall."
-Nelson Mandela

Don't overthink this—like Nike says, Just Do It! Exercise has so many incredible benefits to the human body, but some of the most important benefits to those of us living with diabetes are lower blood sugars, needing less insulin/oral medications, higher energy levels, increased confidence, increased strength, an overall sense of empowerment and wellbeing, and just the feeling of being able to get things done!

1. **Schedule It.** For the next 30 days, the most important thing to concentrate on is getting some movement in on a consistent basis, and the only way that is going to happen is if you schedule it. Putting an appointment in our calendar with a reminder 15 minutes beforehand makes it REAL. The amount of time you schedule when first getting started is not important. Start with ten minutes a day and slowly build from there, being super conscious of not overdoing it or setting goals that are unrealistic for your current level of physical fitness or current frequency of physical activity (aka self-sabotage).

2. **Focus on Form.** Whatever you choose to do, whether it is walking or introducing some bodyweight exercises, the most important thing to focus on is doing it properly. If you are walking, try to concentrate on not letting your shoulders slump forward and keeping your eyes focused ahead so your spine is nice and straight. If you are incorporating any bodyweight exercises, make sure you watch an instructional video about proper form before getting started, or hire a qualified trainer.

3. **Practice Pride.** No matter what you are able to do right now, you must celebrate your efforts and feel proud that you moved at all. There is no amount of exercise that shouldn't be celebrated. Pat yourself on the back and smile big, because you earned it. If you are currently injured, PLEASE talk to your doctor, or preferably your physical therapist, to discuss what options are safe for you at the current time.

4. **Take the Big Blue Test.** Not only is this a great way to really see what just a little bit of exercise can do for our blood sugars and our moods, but this is also a great way to join thousands of other people in the DOC who know the huge impacts that small changes can have on our health. Go to **www.bigbluetest.org** for a fun jumpstart to your fitness journey. By taking a minute to enter a few data points (what your blood sugar was before exercising, and what is was after), not only are you contributing to valuable research and doing wonders for your own health, but you are also donating $1 to charities that provide diabetes supplies to those in need. It doesn't get any easier or more beneficial than that!

According to the Big Blue Test's website via the Diabetes Hands Foundation, "Since 2010, over 40,000 people helped themselves while helping more than 10,000 others. Most participants in the Big Blue Test experience an average blood sugar drop of 20%. Each Big Blue Test helps you and helps others, through a life-saving donation made on your behalf. This has translated in $250,000 awarded by Diabetes Hands Foundation in Big Blue Test grants in the past four years." Having the chance to not only improve our own lives, but to help benefit the lives of others in the process is an amazing opportunity to take advantage of!

I've put together the following list of eight bodyweight exercises that I love, are simple enough to learn, and can all be done from the comfort of our own homes, with absolutely no equipment. A gym membership is not a requirement for being able to exercise!

All of the following exercises can be modified for the beginner to the athlete, for any desired levels of difficulty.

Eight To Dominate Bodyweight Exercises:
Push-up
Downward Dog to High Plank
Low Plank
Low Side Plank
Squat
Glute Bridge/Marching Soldiers
Burpees
Mountain Climbers

I've made short videos, which are all available on my *YouTube* channel, demonstrating proper form for all of the above exercises, and as I've said before, FORM IS EVERYTHING! When it comes to exercise, no matter if it's cardio or resistance training, it is always quality over quantity. Performing repetitions of exercises without proper form can lead to injuries, pulls, strains, sprains, and ultimately training our bodies to move in ways that will hurt us instead of helping us. Please take the time to be sure that you are breathing, and positioning and moving your body correctly, by watching the instructional videos as many times as needed. Working out in front of a mirror and/or recording yourself on your phone can also be helpful tools to review your movements and ensure that you are moving correctly.

Here are a variety of options for different ways/schemes to perform the bodyweight resistance training exercises so you can mix things up any way you like.

| Hypertrophy Training | Pick 3-6 of the exercises and perform 3 sets of 12 reps of each, with 30 seconds of rest between each set. Do each exercise for 3 sets/12 reps and then move on to the next exercise. **Example:** 3 sets/12 |

	reps of push-ups (rest 30 seconds between each set of 12 push-ups), then 30 seconds rest before moving on to 3 sets/12 reps of squats, etc.
5/10/15 Split	Pick 3 of the exercises and perform one for 5 reps, one for 10 reps, and one for 15 reps, which completes one round. Complete as many rounds as you can in 15 minutes, resting when needed. **Example:** 5 push-ups, 10 squats, 15 glute bridges = 1 round. Repeat same sequence for as many rounds as you can in 15 minutes.
Tabata	Pick 3-4 of the exercises and perform them in 3-minute blocks for an intense workout, lasting 12-15 minutes in total. "Tabata" means that you will perform each exercise in 3-minute blocks, using your maximum effort for 20 seconds and then resting for 10 seconds, and then repeating maximum effort for 20 seconds, rest for 10 seconds. This repeats for 3 minutes, which means that you will perform 6 rounds of each exercise during the 3-minute block. **Example:** Squat for 20 seconds, rest for 10 seconds, squat for 20 seconds, rest for 10 seconds (this will complete one minute of the 3-minute block.) Rest for one minute between each 3 minute block of exercise.
Circuit	Choose 4-6 exercises and

	perform as many reps of each exercise as you can in one minute before immediately moving on to the next one. This circuit can be done for 2-6 rounds, depending on your current level of strength and endurance. **Example:** Push-ups for 1 minute, squats for 1 minute, plank for 1 minute, Bird Dogs for 1 minute, which completes one round of a 4-exercise circuit.

No matter what kind of workout you choose to do, it is very important to include at least one day per week (a full 24 hours) of rest, in order for your body to have the proper time to adapt and repair itself (this is where getting enough sleep is a huge factor as well). In addition to the Eight to Dominate exercises, here are some great cardio suggestions. You can do cardio and bodyweight exercises on the same day, or on separate days, or just choose to do one or the other—whatever makes you happy, and that you are willing and able to work into your schedule is most important.

Cardio Options/Examples:
Walk/Jog/Run/Sprint
Rowing Machine/Erg
Swimming
Jump Rope
Elliptical
Bike Riding (stationary bike/spinning/road-biking)
Skipping (yes, I'm totally serious, it's very difficult!)
Zumba

One way to mix things up and maximize results for your time spent when it comes to cardio is to incorporate interval training. You can complete a great interval cardio workout in 20 minutes, and keep burning calories for hours after you are finished. An interval workout consists of work performed at a high level of intensity for a short period of time, then a longer period of recovery, then repeating that cycle. For example, let's say you pick walking/jogging as your cardio. Here is how that might look as interval training:

Warm-up walking: 5 minutes

Jog/run: 15-30 seconds (15 seconds for beginners; 30 seconds for those who are accustomed to working out regularly)

Walk/recover: 60-90 seconds (90 seconds for beginners; 60 seconds for those who are accustomed to working out regularly)

Repeat this interval six or more times, completely depending on how you are feeling and what your current level of physical fitness is. There is no right or wrong amount of times to do this! Once you are able to do that particular interval about ten times, that's when you know you are ready to either increase your intensity during the jog/run portion, increase your time during the jog/run portion, and/or decrease your walk/recover time.

Don't change all of these variables at once! Choose one at a time and go from there. Don't put any expectations on this, other than to get stronger week by week, like increasing your intensity on the jog/run portion, or adding another round to the intervals (if you did five rounds last week, aim for six the next week, etc.) If you do this, you will improve your cardiovascular strength (read: strengthen your heart), increase your lung capacity, decrease your resting heart rate, and increase your overall physical and mental strength and clarity.

You can also choose to do any of these cardio options at a steady state. This means that your aim is to keep your heart rate at roughly 65-75% of your maximum heart rate throughout the whole workout (max heart rate can be found by subtracting your age from 220). For example, my maximum heart rate is 187 beats per minute (bpm) because I am 33 years old, and 220-33 = 187. This means that my steady state zone is between 121-140 bpm. All I did to figure that out was multiply my max heart rate of 187 by 0.65 to get the 65%, and by 0.75 to get the 75% on my computer calculator. I personally prefer a mix of intervals and steady state for variety, but you should do whatever is most appealing and most enjoyable for you! Again, no right or wrong answer!

Yoga

Because of the incredible physical, mental, emotional, and spiritual effects that practicing yoga has had on me and on so many of my friends, family, and clients, I have to say a few words about it here. Before I tried yoga for the first time, I had preconceived notions about it. I thought it was just not for me, but boy was I wrong. Now I know without a shadow of a doubt that yoga is for everyone, and I am not one to make broad generalizations about one single form of physical movement.

Whether you choose cardio, bodyweight exercises, take classes, or any other form of exercise, it's totally your call. But I believe with every fiber of my being that yoga is an essential complement to every other form of exercise that exists. It offers a mind-body connection that is indescribable unless you've experienced it yourself. Yoga comes in many forms, styles, and levels of intensity.

You don't need to do handstands or crazy acts of circus-like balance to experience the incredible benefits of practicing yoga. The simple acts of stretching, moving slowly and deliberately, and quieting our minds in order to pay attention to our bodies offers a level of freedom and sometimes even catharsis that can only be understood through experience. I highly recommend checking out a local beginner's class, or simply finding one of thousands of free yoga classes on *YouTube* and giving it an honest try. It might take a few practices to be able to quiet the mind down enough to truly experience the bliss it offers, but it is worth the effort on all fronts. I can't say enough good things about yoga and the endless mind-body benefits it offers.

The bottom line is, for the next 30 days (and with intention to use the next 30 days to create the habit of exercising regularly for life), move more than you normally do, and have fun with it! Schedule it and concentrate on your form. Use the exercises and instructions above to build workouts that you enjoy and feel confident about performing. Much like nutrition, exercise is not one-size-fits-all. That's why I encourage everyone to try different things to see what they like. And don't be afraid to change it up as often as you want. Whatever you do, make sure you allow yourself to celebrate your achievements and to feel proud, confident, and accomplished when you are done!

22

TAKE ACTION: SUPPORT

"Rather light a candle than complain about darkness."
-Chinese proverb

This section is all about continuing to make strides outside of our comfort zones. It's time to reach out to others, ask for support, and begin to find your favorite places in the DOC (diabetes online community). Head over to **www.diabetesoc.com** and check out all the resources to find blogs, articles, forums, *Facebook* groups, *Twitter* chats, and more. Remember, I just recently started this resource site, and I'm always open to learning about more DOC sites to add. Email me at **Coach@diabetesdomintor.com** with any suggestions!

This is also the section where we make sure that the ways we are supporting ourselves are where we want them to be. Remember, we must be our own best support system, because we believe that we deserve to be well taken care of, and that we deserve the gift of health and self-love. It is time to take the actions that will allow us to get past our beliefs that we are in this alone, because that simply isn't true.

There are millions of us out there going through similar struggles every single day, and once in a while, we all just need to talk to someone who understands. These people won't just magically find you, though. You have to step up (and out of your comfort zone) and reach out. Set yourself up for support success because one day (much sooner than you may think), you will have the opportunity to pay it forward and support someone else who needs to hear your voice, just as you needed to hear theirs. This diabetes journey is not meant to be traveled alone!

1. **Self-Support.** If you are unsatisfied with your doctor, endocrinologist, or any critical member of your healthcare team, now is the time to find a doctor/healthcare professional who you like, if you have insurance that allows you to choose from a certain pool of doctors who are "in

network." If this is not an option, put together a list of concerns that you have, and have an open discussion with your current doctor the next time you see him or her. Sometimes doctors are so busy and have a lot of pressure on them to make appointments go quickly, so hearing your concerns about not feeling like your needs as a patient are being satisfied, along with clear suggestions on what you think can be done to solve the issue could really turn things around on the next visit and moving forward. We must have a healthcare team that treats us like human beings, and not walking chronic illnesses.

I found my current endocrinologist from a recommendation from my Omnipod sales/training rep. I enjoy and recommend getting recommendations from other people. If you haven't had your A1c checked within the past 3-4 months, make an appointment to get it done, as well as a full lipid panel (cholesterol) so you know where you are now, which will allow you to more intelligently decide exactly where you want to go. If you do have health insurance and aren't sure if it will cover items such as CGMs or insulin pumps, and you are interested in learning more, you must call your insurance company to find out, or call Dexcom or the pump company you are considering who very well may do the work for you. By limiting your technological support based on the simple fact that you just don't know what your options are and haven't taken the time to investigate, you limit how far you can go and how much you can continue to improve.

If you are lacking enough of any of the diabetes supplies you need to take the best possible care of yourself, this is the time to follow some (or all) of the suggestions from the "Support" section above. Talk to your doctor about needing more supplies, and see if they can provide you with some samples or if they have any other recommendations. Go to your local walk-in clinic and explain the situation to them to see if they can help or offer further suggestions. Contact the manufacturer of whatever it is you need more of (insulin, test strips, etc.), and see if they have programs for those who cannot afford enough supplies. Seek out and join any number of *Facebook* groups (Type 1 Diabetic's Pay It Forward, and Pay It Forward Diabetes US Only are two examples of many groups like this, more available on **www.diabetesoc.com**) and see if you can work out a barter, or if someone has what you need and can send it to you for the cost of shipping.

There are other options, such as buying a store brand meter (CVS, Rite Aid, Walgreens, or Walmart, to name a few), which offer test strips at a much more affordable price than name-brand meter test strips. There is also a new company called Livongo Health that offers a high-tech meter and unlimited test strips for a monthly fee. My point is that there are many options, and unless we believe we are worth it and are willing to take the time to take the ACTIONS to explore these options, we will never know what is really available to us. We must love ourselves enough to reach out for help when we need it so that we have the ability to take the best care of ourselves as possible since it is ultimately our job, and most likely nobody is going to do it for us.

Finally, support yourself by setting alarms or reminders on your cellphone for anything that you know you regularly forget to do, such as checking your blood sugar or taking insulin or medication at specific times. Don't let something as simple (and avoidable) as planning ahead continually trip you up!

2. **Friends and Family.** If you are in a situation where you rarely ever talk about your diabetes with anyone in your group of friends, family, co-workers, etc., and you feel like having an open dialogue with one or more of those people could really make communications between everyone better, now is the time to reach out to them. A good way to go about this is to sit down and make a list of what you might want to talk about and why. Knowing what outcomes you are after and being able to clearly communicate those desired outcomes to the people we reach out to can make all the

difference in the world. It also allows us to approach them in a less emotionally charged state, which for many reasons can produce more progress-oriented outcomes.

I'm not saying you can't be emotional about your diabetes or that you should stifle emotions, but when approaching someone who might not understand your day-to-day life, it can be more productive to be clear about what you hope to achieve by opening up this dialogue. Maybe you want them to better understand the mood swings that happen with low and high blood sugars. Maybe you want them to better understand how much constant work you put in to your diabetes care, since most people don't see all that you do.

Maybe you want them to know that you are trying your best and that sometimes, you just need a hug. You might be surprised to find that the people you reach out to also very much wanted to open up a productive dialogue with you, but didn't know how to best approach it. Reaching out for help can be an immensely gratifying learning and growing experience for all parties involved, and can bring the relationships we have with those people much closer together.

3. **DOC (diabetes online community).** Get in where you fit in. When it comes to the DOC, there are unlimited options to find where you feel most comfortable. No matter what type of diabetes you have, there are multiple *Facebook* groups created just for your type. If you are an athlete with diabetes, there are *Facebook* groups for that. No matter what nutritional lifestyle you choose to follow, there is a *Facebook* group for that as well. No matter what pump or CGM you might use, there are multiple groups for all of them. If you are on MDI (manual daily injections), there are groups for that too. It is up to you to find and join these groups, which is the easy part. Then you must speak up and start a dialogue in those groups to see who else is out there and going through what you are currently dealing with. Many times, we take the

conversations that started in a thread in a *Facebook* group to the more private option of instant messaging.

From there, I know that both I and many other members of the DOC have created instant bonds and lasting friendships with other people living with diabetes who just get us. The thing is, if you never put yourself out there, you will never know what amazing connections and friendships you are missing out on.

The most popular and accessible online forum that is running 24/7 is **www.tudiabetes.org.** You can create an account and login anytime to join a variety of existing conversations about all things regarding life with diabetes. If you like *Twitter*, every Wednesday night at 9pm Eastern Time, there is a live chat between members of the DOC on a wide variety of topics. Using the hashtag #DSMA (which stands for Diabetes Social Media Advocacy), you have the opportunity to join an ongoing conversation about living with diabetes with people from all over the world. There is also another awesome Twitter chat that follows the hashtag #DCDE (which stands for Diabetic Connect Diabetes Education) that happens every Tuesday night at 9pm Eastern Time.

These are just a few suggestions, and the opportunities to join the DOC in some way are pretty much endless. There is no excuse to go through this alone, because you are never alone unless you choose to isolate yourself from your peers who are always waiting to welcome you in the DOC with open arms. The benefits of getting involved with the DOC are vast. The feeling of belonging to a group of people who always know what you are talking about is an incredible feeling. Being able to learn from others' experiences, and having the ability to integrate those lessons into our own lives is invaluable.

Always having someone cheering you on, or to have a group of people to celebrate (or commiserate) your latest A1c reading with can make all the difference in the world. People always rooting you on to win, and people with whom to celebrate those wins when you reach them is what the DOC provides. And you already know how I feel about the importance of celebrating!

Even if you are shy or hesitant to interact on any of these sites, it is so helpful and uplifting to just go and observe what is going on. You will still have the opportunity to learn so much even if you choose to stay quiet at first. Take it one step at a time and go at your own pace. The important thing is to take the first step and simply log on!

We have so many options available to us in the way of support today, from loving ourselves, to family and friends, to doctors and nutritionists, to various machines, and to an endless network of peer love and support, but it's up to us to take the actions necessary to make sure we get the support we need. Set yourself up for success. Start making yourself a little network, even if it's just you right now.

Everyone has to start somewhere, and the key is not to give up, no matter how many times we fall. The only time we fail is when we stop trying. Everything that happens before you succeed that you perceive as failure is just experience and lessons learned; and the more experience we have, the more informed our decisions can be moving forward.

23

TAKE ACTION: BODY SYSTEMS

"Success is nothing more than a few simple disciplines, practiced every day."
-Jim Rohn

This is the only section where I included the "Take Action" items in the previous section, since everything involved is pretty straightforward. I am going to copy and paste them here in order to keep up with consistency, and so you don't have to go searching for the things that need to get done in another section, but they are the same recommendations from Part Two. When we sleep, our bodies have time to heal and adapt, and that is something that every single one of us needs every single day. If we want to reach a new level with our health, we need to ensure that we are getting a minimum of seven solid hours of sleep per night, but preferably eight, or even nine.

Changes don't happen unless we make changes to our actions. Commit to making your health a top priority in order to present the best version of yourself that you can be to everyone in your life. Doing this will help to create better communication, better quality of relationships, and an overall feeling of being well-rested and ready to handle whatever each day brings with less feelings of stress.

1. **Black-out curtains, and blacking out all of the lights in the room.** This includes alarm clocks, lights coming from cellphone chargers, and literally every speck of light. I'm talking pitch-black-can't-see-your-hand-in-front-of-your-face dark. I have black trash bags over my bedroom windows so I can enjoy the deep sleep that a pitch-black room provides. No shame in my sleep game! They sell black-out curtains at places like Walmart and K-Mart, which are very affordable.

2. **De-screening.** This is one that most of us have probably heard is helpful, but may not have been able to exert the self-control to try yet. Consciously choosing to turn off access to

ALL screens 30-60 minutes before bed allows our brains to settle into a restful state. When we have the lights from a screen shining into our eyes, it signals to our brains that it's time to be active, which is the exact opposite of what we need to settle into a restful sleep. Everything on social media will be there in the morning, and your sleep is much more important than anyone's status update!

3. **Bedtime yoga.** I know, at first, it might sound counter-productive to do anything physical before going to bed, but gentle stretching can release relaxing hormones into our systems that allow us to more easily calm down, both physically and mentally. There are countless bedtime yoga routines on *YouTube* to choose from. Doing this before bed also allows us to get out of our heads and slow down the chatter. Many of the bedtime yoga routines are designed to actually be done in bed. I realize this will require some use of a screen at first, but eventually, you will learn the stretches and can just listen to the prompts instead of staring at the screen the whole time.

4. **Meditation.** Other than the black-out curtains, this is my favorite helper, and one that I've found to be incredibly effective in helping to stop the seemingly inevitable mind-racing that pops up as soon as I lie down. Again, there are a multitude of guided meditations for sleep on *YouTube*; it's just a matter of finding one that you enjoy. I use an app on my phone called "The Oprah & Deepak 21-Day Meditation Experience." I like these because they are short (20 minutes) and meaningful, and truly allow my brain to focus on drifting off, rather than on the million things that I need to get done in my life!

5. **Sleep-inducing background noise.** I know that the word "noise" in itself might sound like something that wouldn't help us sleep, but depending on the type of noise, it can be super helpful. I personally turn on the sound of a fireplace after I finish with my meditation, through an app called "Sleep Pillow," and there are many other sleep-noise apps available. Some of us might like the sound of the ocean, while others might prefer the sound of rain, and some of us might not like any sounds at all—we are all different! Once you find

what you like, it can make a huge difference in your ability to fall and stay asleep.

6. **Not having a full stomach.** Trying to fall asleep with a stomach full of food can definitely make things more difficult. Digestion is a process that will always come first in the human body. If there is food to be digested, the body will get to work on digesting it, instead of focusing on falling asleep. If you feel hungry before bed, I recommend having a small portion of something that is very quickly digested, like fruits or vegetables. Aim to eat dinner, at the very least, 2-3 hours before going to bed to get as restful a night's sleep as possible.

Here is a quick recap of how to make sure we poop every single day, and ideally, more than once per day. It is one of the worst feelings to be bloated, to have our stomachs distended and to feel uncomfortable because we are unable to rid our bodies of waste. I can't stress enough how crucial this is to our overall health and well-being. Do not let another day go by before incorporating these actions into your daily routine in order to reset your body and to begin eliminating on a consistent basis.

1. **Choose to be Properly Hydrated All of the Time.** I realize that at this point I might sound like a broken record, but drinking a minimum of our bodyweight in ounces of water per day can be the only thing missing from being on a regular elimination schedule. Three-quarters of an average, healthy poop is made up of water. When constipated, waste materials stay in the large intestine longer and more water is removed causing the feces to become hard and difficult to pass. So drink up!

2. **Eat More Fiber.** It becomes easier to get enough fiber in our diets once we begin focusing on a whole foods, nutrient dense way of eating. Lots of vegetables, fruits, beans, nuts, and seeds will all do the trick. Some of the higher fiber items are avocados, peas, all leafy greens, squash, sweet potatoes, pears, all berries, chia seeds, flax seeds, apples, oranges, prunes, all beans, and quinoa. These are just a few of the

endless options for filling up our diets with fiber-rich foods. I recommend aiming for 30-40 grams of fiber per day.

3. **Get Moving to Get Things Moving.** Once you begin exercising, sometimes that is all it takes to begin eliminating regularly. Seems simple enough, I know. But sometimes all it takes to get things moving, is, well, to get moving!

4. **Supplements.** I highly recommend trying all of the above options first before adding in supplements, but if you've been trying consistently for over a week, using the first 3 options and are not seeing any results, adding in a fiber supplement could do the trick. Some options that I recommend are Garden of Life RAW Organic Fiber, Organic Triple Fiber by Renew Life, or Optimum Nutrition Fitness Fiber, all of which can be found on *Amazon* and other online retailers. Please be sure to stay well hydrated when taking any fiber supplements!

24

TAKE ACTION: MINDFULNESS

"The more you praise and celebrate your life, the more there is in life to celebrate."
-Oprah Winfrey

As I've mentioned before, all of the six pillars are very closely related to one another. Often, the actions we take in order to achieve a higher level of mastery in one of the pillars will cause us to achieve a higher level of mastery in some (or all) of the others. This is an example of a welcomed domino effect, or what I like to call an upward spiral.

When it comes to mindfulness, there are a few actions that, if we commit to taking each day, will allow us to be so much more present on a consistent basis in our day-to-day lives, not only with our own health, but with our interactions with others as well. Mindfulness is the key to improving our relationships with ourselves, which in turn improves the way we relate to others throughout all aspects of life. It's a win/win situation!

1. **Check in.** Set recurring reminders on your phone for three different times throughout each day. I like to check in with myself first thing in the morning, mid-afternoon, and later in the evening. What I mean by "check in" is to become fully present with ourselves. During those few minutes when we are tuning in, we intentionally focus our awareness on the signs our bodies are sending us. What signs are our bodies sending us? How are we feeling? What is our mood like? To make it simple, use a scale of one to ten, where one means you are literally ripping your hair out and can't function at all, and ten means you feel incredibly good and you are happy beyond measure.

   If you are under a five or six, ask yourself a productive question such as, "What can I do right now to improve my mood?" With all of the skills you learned above, you know right away that you could take a few minutes to practice gratitude stacking, or you could take a quick walk around the block, among other things. We have so many tools that are always available to us that will help us change our mood instantly. It is up to us to take (schedule) the time to be present and check in, and to intentionally use these tools to actively shape our realities.

2. **Know your outcome and be intentional.** One of the most helpful aspects of practicing mindfulness is to know, very specifically, what outcome you are after before going into any situation or conversation. This applies quite literally to every single thing we ever do, from a doctor's appointment, to a conversation with our child's teacher, to reading an article online, to checking our blood sugar. What do we want to achieve by participating in this experience? What do we want to contribute to or gain from this interaction?

    When we intentionally choose to identify and be aware of what we want beforehand, we are much more likely to actually get it, whatever it is. If we intentionally say that the desired outcome of checking our blood sugar is to simply know what is going on inside of our bodies right now so we can make an informed decision about what actions to take next, then the results of that check can and will be much less likely to cause us to feel negative emotions if the results are out of the range for which we are aiming.

    By knowing our desired outcomes and intentionally expressing them to ourselves and the universe, we instantly become more objective and less judgmental (of ourselves and others), no matter what the situation. Knowing our outcomes and being intentional about the outcomes we choose to pursue are powerful ways to be more in control of the way we feel and the mindsets we have about pretty much every situation in life.

3. **Don't let "I Already Know That Syndrome" ruin your willingness to be present.** The next time you are at the doctor, or at a conference, or anywhere where someone is

talking or teaching about an area of health or life about which you think you already know everything, don't immediately tune-out. Instead, stop and do a quick assessment of the situation. If your doctor/CDE/nutritionist or the speaker at the conference is talking about pre-bolusing for meals, for example, instead of just thinking or saying, "I already know that" and going for your cellphone, take a moment to ask yourself if that is something that you are habitually and consistently doing in your life. If it is, then it's all good and move on. But if it's not, catch yourself in the act.

Kindly and without judgment, say to yourself that even though you are aware that pre-bolusing for meals is important to mitigate post-meal blood sugar spikes and can make a big difference in overall A1c readings, you are not currently practicing it. Choose to remain present in the conversation instead of being instantly dismissive because you believe you already know something. Choose to remain mindful of the fact that there might be something new to learn, or a way you might be able to benefit from hearing this information again. Remember, repetition is the mother of skill.

4. **Put the phone down.** Make it a priority on your path to living more mindfully to put your phone down more often. Disconnect from the screen and re-connect with everything that is going on around you. Reconnect with your dreams and desires and the things you want out of life. Don't allow someone with whom you are interacting to be a victim of your "digital disrespect." Choose to be fully present.

When you are walking in public, intentionally put your phone away and resist the urge to look at it. Instead, notice other people. Smile at them, interact with them. Delete certain apps from your phone in order to be more present in life. If you know you habitually check *Facebook, Twitter, Instagram, YouTube*, your email, or any other online site multiple times every day, eliminate the app and lessen your ability to disconnect from the real world.

Choose to take back control of your schedule, and not to be at the whims of whomever is trying to get your attention via email or social media. Schedule specific times each day (once in the morning after your morning routine, and once in the evening, for example) when you dedicate those few minutes to checking your email and looking at social media, and make sure that scheduled time has a specific end so you don't get caught up and lose countless hours out of your day.

When we are constantly buried in our phones, we are actively choosing to allow other people to rule our schedules and lives. We are saying that other people's agendas are more important than our own, and that we are committing to responding to their wants and needs before our own. This is a power that many of us are actively giving up every single day, and one that we must reclaim in order to have the mental bandwidth to focus on our own hopes and dreams, our own passions in life, our own health and well-being. Choose to put the phone down and reclaim your day!

25

CALL TO ACTION!

I am not a product of my circumstances. I am a product of my decisions."
Stephen Covey

"Never limit the vision you have for your life based on your current circumstances or competencies."
-Brendon Burchard

Trusting Your "True You"

I've given you a lot of information in this book. I genuinely hope that you have become inspired to step up to the challenge of embracing the Diabetes Dominator mentality in order to liberate yourself from the negativity and uncertainty that can be a part of managing life with diabetes. This book is designed to help the reader create sustainable healthy habits, which evolve into a sustainable healthy lifestyle.

You can do this. And the reason I know that you can do this is because I did this WITHOUT this guide! That alone lets us know that it's possible. I have helped many clients gain confidence and to own their expertise in managing their diabetes, and they all had one very important thing in common: a strong desire to change the current status of their health and their relationship with diabetes.

If we want something bad enough, there is nothing that can stand in our way. Perfection is not what we are after. The main focus is consistently getting a little bit healthier with your choices each day, focusing on continuous progress. The only way that we can truly fail at any endeavor in life is if we give up and don't keep trying. Falling down is part of the journey, the most important part is standing back up every time.

If you've read this entire book, you know more about diabetes management than the majority of people with diabetes in the world. Own your expertise, and put it into practice. There is nobody more qualified to manage your diabetes day-to-day that you.

Maybe your practice will influence others to want to choose to lead a healthier lifestyle. When I first began focusing on taking control of my choices and building a healthy lifestyle, influencing others was not something that I thought about. But now it is my biggest motivator to continue leading by example. Change is good. And if you run into another person with diabetes that needs some help, reach out and be supportive. The more we willingly and openly share our stories and experiences with others, the more support and love we build in our diabetes community.

I'm a huge fan of, and believer in the saying "when the student is ready, the teacher will appear." This has rung true for me on so many occasions in my life that I don't know if simple coincidence can explain it. There is some reason why you are reading these words right now. I don't know what it is, but don't ignore the signs that are right in front of you, the signs that the universe is sending you, not only now, but always.

Happiness begins with our health. You have a step by step guide to take control of your health-related choices in your hands right now. Coincidence? Open your mind and your heart to what is possible, and you will find that the possibilities will open up to you. Be open to love, learning, action, growth, contribution, and change, and trust your logic and common sense.

We live in a world that is constantly changing, and the desire to be in control of our lives drives almost all of us. The one thing I've found throughout my many years of fighting to stay "in control" of my life is that the only thing that we as human beings truly do have control over are our choices. What we do and don't eat, how we do or don't move, and the attitudes we choose to project out into the world.

Once we have that control over our choices, the feelings of self-love, confidence, and empowerment spill over into all other areas of our lives. Choose to step up and take control of your choices, it will be the best decision you've ever made, both for yourself and for everyone that you love and that loves you. The best project you will ever work on is you. The best investment you can ever make is in your own personal development. Now is always the best time to create a sustainable healthy lifestyle. Stand back up no matter how many times you fall, and no matter how long it might take to get back up.

If you would like to go further with your training and your improvement, then I have a $47 video training series on the 6 Pillars of Total Health that I would like to offer you for free for reading this book, and committing to taking action on improving your health and your relationship with diabetes. Go to **diabetesdominator.com/freetraining** to sign up!

PART FIVE - DIABETES DOMINATOR INTERVIEWS

INTERVIEWS WITH DIABETES DOMINATORS THRIVING WITH DIABETES

ASHA BROWN

Question 1: Who are you? What makes you happy? What hobbies are you passionate about? Who do you love? What do you do for a living? Essentially, your bio plus some personal stuff!

My name is Asha Brown and I am the Founder and Executive Director of We Are Diabetes, a nonprofit organization primarily devoted to supporting type one diabetics who struggle with eating disorders and other co-occurring mental health concerns. Cats make me very happy; so do gluten free corn dogs with lots of ketchup! I also get a really big thrill out of crossing things off of a "to-do" list and learning new things.

I'm passionate about helping others rediscover who they are, beyond their type one diabetes, and beyond their eating disorders! I'm also passionate about living well, and living fully. Sometimes that means walking a very different path than what is considered "normal", but I've learned that the most important thing in life is to stay true to yourself. I love yoga, being awake before everyone else, sweet potatoes, coconut oil, and thrift shopping. I love my family and my husband, and I love my diabetes community.

Question 2: What is your diabetes story? Please share your story of diagnosis and the path you traveled to get where you are today. What have been your biggest struggles/triumphs in regard to living with diabetes? How does diabetes makes you awesome at life? What are the tools you use to manage your diabetes day to day (pump, MDI, CGM, etc.)?

I was diagnosed with type one diabetes when I was five years old. My dad also has type one diabetes (he was diagnosed in 1970) so I didn't have a very dramatic entrance in to my new life as a T1D; I just started taking shots and testing my blood sugar just like my dad did.

My chronic illness didn't get in my way of having a joyful childhood, but by the time I was a freshman in high school things had changed dramatically. I was tired of carrying my diabetes supplies around with me, tired of having to eat a snack when other people were able to continue on with their day and just eat when they were actually hungry.

Along with my T1D diagnosis at age five, I was diagnosed with hypothyroid at age 8, and later on I was diagnosed PCOS (Polycystic Ovary Syndrome) at age 16. I started to feel like I was broken, and started to resent having to always deal with my diabetes. I also started to get upset at all the poorly written information about diabetes that I was reading in magazines and books. I kept reading that a person with all of my chronic conditions tended to be overweight, and was doomed to always having trouble managing a healthy weight. That's not what a 16 year old girl living in a thin-obsessed culture wants or needs to hear over and over again.

I remember feeling outraged; I hadn't done anything to deserve a life-sentence of living in a body that wasn't my own to control. As a performer, and a professional actress since childhood, I remember making a promise to myself that I would never let diabetes get in the way of my dreams of a life on the stage. I started to take less insulin in order to avoid having any possibility of low blood sugars during rehearsals or while performing. Knowing that there was no way I could go low soothed the anxiety I was starting to develop about my diabetes, so I continued to keep my blood sugars elevated. It really went downhill from there.

What continued from this point was a decade long journey in to a deadly eating disorder that I meticulously hid from everyone, even my dad. I spent a decade of my life lying to everyone, and hating myself. I tried many times to pull myself out of the dark hole I had created, but I had no idea how to live without my eating disorder. It had become who I was, and it dictated every decision I made. It wasn't until I fell in love and got married that I had the courage to fight for my freedom.

I've been given a second chance at life. Unfortunately there are many like me who aren't as lucky. It's devastating to know how many diabetics are struggling with an eating disorder, without support or educated providers to guide them towards recovery. Ironically, my biggest struggle with my diabetes has transformed in to my biggest triumph. All of the energy and commitment that was being used to "maintain" my eating disorder has been redirected towards We Are Diabetes.

WAD was not a quick decision. The first two years of my recovery were devoted to learning how to function in the real world, without the security blanket of my all-consuming obsession. As I regained my spirit, I realized that no one was talking about diabetes and eating disorders. The amount of credible support I found online was disheartening to say the least, and I felt a stir inside my soul that whispered: "you have to do this". I took my time, I did my research, and I made sure that my recovery was rock solid before I started giving advice and guidance to others. Once the We Are Diabetes website was launched in January 2012, we hit the ground running!

I didn't expect to be running a nonprofit, nor did I expect my life to be devoted to diabetes advocacy. I'd told myself ever since I was cast in my first film at age five that I was going to be an actress. However, the work I do now is more satisfying than a thousand standing ovations. I'm eternally grateful to have the opportunity to support others, and to show them that there is a way "out" of the exhausting cycle of living with diabetes and an eating disorder.

As for managing my diabetes, I love, love, LOVE my Dexcom CGM. It took me a long time to get over my angst at having a device attached to my body 24/7, but I'm so grateful for all my T1D friends who helped me conquer my hang-ups and take the plunge. My dad was so impressed with my Dexcom that he immediately got one of his own. It makes me so happy that now I can celebrate diabetes triumphs with one of the most important men in my life, instead of keeping secrets. Also I'm on MDI (manual daily injections) and proud of it!

Question 3: What are your top 3 tips for thriving with diabetes that you believe have served you (and continue to serve you) best along your diabetes journey?

1. Embrace the fact that you will always have a bigger purse, or man-satchel.

I'm sure I look like a college student to most people because I carry a backpack with me everywhere I go. I can sometimes be out of the house from 6am to 7pm, and I would prefer to have extra supplies and enough snacks for multiple lows, (or "almost lows") then have to shell out extra money for unhealthy substitutes. I have a lot less anxiety leaving the house for a long day knowing I have back up testing supplies and CGM tape tucked away, as well as a few healthy snacks in case I don't make it home for a while for a proper meal. Of course I love the idea of just having a small handbag to carry with me during the day, but it's not realistic for my lifestyle. The reason I thrive with T1D is because I embrace the fact that I need a lot of stuff for my diabetes during the day. Instead of being in denial about it, I welcome it with a sense of creativity; I try to pick out fun colored backpacks whenever I treat myself to a new one.

2. If it's something you can do in less than a minute you should just do it.

Sometimes I'm just not in the mood to restock my backpack supplies, or check on my insulin inventory in the fridge, but it takes less than 30 seconds, and those 30 seconds will inevitably save me a lot of anxiety and stress down the road. It can be annoying, but it's always better than realizing I've run out of low supplies when I'm out and about, or running out of a prescription instead of taking the minute to refill it.

3. Devote a part of your day to something that has nothing to do with diabetes.

We are not robots, and even though it's important to embrace that T1D requires dedication and acceptance, we are not our chronic illness. I have a very dedicated yoga practice that keeps me sane, and my studio is where I can just "be" no matter what direction my Dexcom arrow is pointing, or what ridiculous scenario my insurance provider is trying to pull. You have to separate yourself from the never ending task of managing this beast once in a while, just enough to remember you are a person, not a machine.

www.wearediabetes.org

SHERI COLBERG

Question 1: Who are you? What makes you happy? What hobbies are you passionate about? Who do you love? What do you do for a living? Essentially, your bio plus some personal stuff!

My name is Sheri Colberg. I was always active as a kid, playing in the woods, building forts, swimming, and just being a tomboy. As a preteen, I began exercising regularly on my own and through organized sports teams because being active was the only thing that gave me any control over my blood glucose levels way back in the "dark ages" of diabetes (before blood glucose meters). I instinctively knew by the way I felt physically after workouts that exercise helped lower my blood glucose into a more normal range and keep it there.

To this day, I still exercise six to seven days a week, just like I started doing regularly almost 40 years ago. I look forward to my daily workouts, vary them to keep working out fun and to keep myself injury-free, and lament the days I am forced to be less physically active. When people ask me how I manage to juggle a full-time career, a happy marriage, and three sons, I tell them simply, "I work out." It gives me the endurance to do everything I need to get done in a day.

Learning why exercise is so beneficial when it comes to diabetes can be very motivating. Due to its positive effect on metabolism, exercise can virtually "erase" overeating mistakes and keep you from getting other health problems like heart disease. Diabetes has been a positive, shaping force in my life when it comes to physical activity in general. I fully embrace it and use diabetes as an excuse to put my workouts first!

I'm also in excellent health because of my lifestyle choices, despite having diabetes for almost five decades. Diabetes gave me an early calling as a healthy lifestyle expert. When I was about 12, I spent a week with my grandmother, who had "borderline" type 2 diabetes. That week, she was on yet another diet, and I decided to help her with dieting—sort of like a wellness coach. I weighed her every morning, measured out her food, and made her run laps around the backyard. We had made a deal that she would pay me $1 for every pound she lost that week with my help, and she lost eight—was I ever a rich kid!

What drove me to become an exercise physiologist, a diabetes researcher, and a college professor was a desire to reach the health goals that I set for myself. After seeing my grandmother suffer through most of the cardiovascular complications associated with uncontrolled diabetes, my focus has been on how to stay healthy with diabetes to order to avoid complications and maintain quality of life. I read about all the horrible things that diabetes was potentially going to do to me when I was in high school and secretly believed that I was going to die before I got a chance to go to college. Since I graduated from high school in 1981, I have made it quite a bit longer than I expected!

You would think that focusing my professional life and career on diabetes and exercise would lead me to constantly be thinking about my own condition, but that is not the case. In my own life, diabetes is in the background. I stop what I'm doing now and then to treat a low or test my blood glucose to maintain control, but rarely give it any thought beyond that.

On a professional level, I have authored 10 books, 16 book chapters, and over 275 articles (**www.SheriColberg.com**), but it all pales in comparison to delivering and raising three healthy sons! I'm on a crusade to help the world live a healthier life (not just a longer one), especially given the current, astronomical rise in the number of cases of all types of diabetes. I have given hundreds of lectures to community and professional audiences around the world with the hope that more knowledge about diabetes will empower people to take better control of their choices and perhaps help prevent type 2.

Truly, it's all about living well while you are alive because without our health, we have nothing. That's why I preach about how important a healthy lifestyle is to maintaining your *quality of life* (whether you have diabetes or not), and that longevity without health is not necessarily a good thing. It's also why I founded a web site (**www.DiabetesMotion.com**) to help everyone with diabetes of any type or prediabetes to exercise safely and effectively.

Question 2: What is your diabetes story? Please share your story of diagnosis and the path you traveled to get where you are today. What have been your biggest struggles/triumphs in regard to living with diabetes? How does diabetes makes you awesome at life? What are the tools you use to manage your diabetes day to day (pump, MDI, CGM, etc.)?

It is hard to even imagine life without diabetes when you get it at the age of four. I really don't remember much about being diagnosed; I just recall feeling kind of sluggish and tired all the time and moping around.

I will be the first one to admit that having diabetes has, in many ways, been a blessing. It likely had a positive impact on my family's overall health, mainly because my mother made the decision that all four of us (my parents, my older brother, and me) would eat the same diabetes diet that was prescribed for me at the time—which included a balanced diet of carbohydrates, protein, and fat, lots of vegetables and fruits, and very limited intake of sweets and refined foods.

What bothered me the most about diabetes at the age of four was not the daily shots, but that I had to give up my favorite cereal, Froot Loops, which contained too much sugar to be on my prescribed "diabetic diet." Even though now I could take a shot of rapid-acting insulin to cover it, you couldn't pay me enough to eat it—yuck! So, did I miss out on having a "normal" childhood filled with sugary cereals, cake, candy, ice cream, and other sweets because of diabetes? Honestly, I don't think so. Personally, I have no problem passing up rich desserts, doughnuts, and other "treats" since I would rather just have a bowl of plain berries. What and when I eat are not dictated by my diabetes, however. I eat when I'm hungry, and I eat healthy foods most of the time because I like them better.

The personal accomplishment that I am most proud of is bearing three healthy sons despite having diabetes. I researched my chances of passing along type 1 diabetes before getting pregnant and enrolled in a research study that allowed me to optimize my control *before* I ever got pregnant with my first child. I never had any problems related to diabetes during my three pregnancies, and I was able to keep my blood glucose under immaculate control throughout. I even exercised throughout all of my pregnancies, which helped with my blood glucose control, and enjoyed having a faster delivery and postpartum recovery. Breastfeeding my three sons for as long as possible also helped with my blood glucose control and with post-pregnancy weight loss, and as an added bonus, it lowered my sons' chances of developing type 1 diabetes themselves. Due to my diabetes, my children have a much healthier diet than most Americans, and they have grown into healthy and active young men.

As far as struggling with diabetes, I have only felt that way on two other occasions in over 47 years with it. One time was when I got my first blood glucose meter in my mid-twenties and had to fully face that I actually have diabetes. (What a revelation after 20 years with it, right?) I think that getting it at the age of four kept me from dealing with it psychologically until I was older and finally had tools to try to more effectively control it.

I felt frustrated while attempting to get a handle on my blood glucose. In the early years (pre-meters), I did the best that I could, but I never really knew what my blood glucose was doing and could not do anything to lower it when I could feel that it was too high—except for exercising. When I finally got a meter while attending a diabetes camp (as an adult collecting data for my first research study), I found out that it was harder to control than I thought. For years I wrote down every morsel of food that I ate, drop of fluid that I drank, and every activity or event in my life in order to figure out the effects of various foods, drinks, and activities.

Honestly, I'm happy to be able to be able to test my blood glucose whenever I want to after years of having no way of knowing exactly what it was! I have tried continuous glucose monitoring as well, but the sensors never seem to calibrate well for me personally, and I have just stuck with meters. I'm low tech with my insulin delivery (syringes and pens), although I have used insulin pumps in the past. My experience is that you still have to be smarter than your pump, and I don't like being without basal insulin if my pump site goes bad.

The other time I struggled with diabetes was when I developed diabetic retinopathy. Ironically, I likely brought it on myself by going from the worst diabetes control of my life (the couple of years before I got my first meter) to the best control very rapidly, which apparently can precipitate its onset. I was only 24 when I saw the first telltale bleed inside my eye, and I soon faced the prospect of going blind for the rest of my life. I underwent a series of laser treatments over the course of two years while my eyes were unstable. I was regularly, but unpredictably, having bleeds into the vitreous fluid inside my eyes that would block my vision for days or weeks at a time. I definitely struggled for a while; I took my biochemistry exam for my PhD program with sight in only one eye and I was legally blind for several weeks after having almost simultaneous bleeds in both eyes. I kept pushing my way through it and never gave up my belief that things would get better. My eyes have now been stable since 1990. I still have problems with night and peripheral vision due to the almost total obliteration of my peripheral retina by the laser treatments, but it's a small price to pay to have my central vision intact.

Question 3: What are your top 3 tips for thriving with diabetes that you believe have served you (and continue to serve you) best along your diabetes journey?

Live life first, and have diabetes second. Don't let having diabetes define you. Live your life and manage your diabetes so you can do everything you want to.

Keep everything in perspective. Although it's not always easy, diabetes is a manageable disease, and you can live a long and healthy life despite having it.

Be grateful for the gifts you have been given, including diabetes. Overcoming obstacles makes you who you are, and managing diabetes can make you a stronger (and, ironically, healthier) person.

Question 4: Is there anything else you would like to share that you think will add value to the readers?

I flirted with the idea of becoming a medical doctor for a while, but after spending some time volunteering in a hospital, I decided that I hated being around sick people in hospitals. That ruled out medical school for me. What I decided to do instead was diabetes research to help cure it. While I have not found the final cure for diabetes or a way to prevent all of its complications, I firmly believe that regular physical activity is about as close to a cure as you can come right now, especially when coupled with a healthy diet and a positive attitude.

You can find Sheri's books online:

Diabetic Athlete's Handbook

Exercise and Diabetes

The Diabetes Break-Through

50 Secrets of the Longest Living People with Diabetes

The 7 Step Diabetes Fitness Plan

www.SheriColberg.com

www.DiabetesMotion.com

Daniele Hargenrader

DIABETIC DANICA

Question 1: Who are you? What makes you happy? What hobbies are you passionate about? Who do you love? What do you do for a living? Essentially, your bio plus some personal stuff!

Hi there! My name is Danica. I'm 23 years old, and my favorite people, sunshine, and coffee make me happy! But, before this gets to sounding like an online dating profile, let's focus more on the main information about me. I just recently entered the "real world", as I graduated in July of 2015 with my second Bachelor's degree. My first degree is in Human Development and Family Sciences, and shortly after that I began an accelerated nursing program to earn my Nursing degree in 13 months! That was probably the second hardest thing I've ever done. The first was being diagnosed with Type 1 diabetes at the age of eleven, but I'll get to that in due time. My ultimate career goal is to become a Certified Diabetes Educator, but as I work towards meeting the qualifications to become a CDE, I am about to begin a job as a pediatric nurse. I have always loved working with kids, and I hope to educate children about their diabetes for my career someday. In the meantime, I also have a YouTube channel called "DiabeticDanica" where I make informative yet entertaining videos about all things diabetes! The channel has just surpassed 10,000 subscribers, and has given me such an amazing avenue to connect with other diabetics online! I am so thankful to have this network of people with diabetes to turn to through the ups and downs of this disease, and to have this creative outlet in which to practice educating about diabetes.

Question 2: What is your diabetes story? Please share your story of diagnosis and the path you traveled to get where you are

today. What have been your biggest struggles/triumphs in regard to living with diabetes? How does diabetes makes you awesome at life? What are the tools you use to manage your diabetes day to day (pump, MDI, CGM, etc.)?

As previously stated, I was diagnosed with Type 1 diabetes at the age of eleven. I was in the park one summer evening with my family listening to an outdoor concert. When I went to use the restroom at the park, something terrifying happened. Well, terrifying to eleven-year-old me at least! I got locked in the bathroom. I distinctly remember being inside the bathroom, flipping the lock open, and grabbing the door handle to turn it, but then the motion of turning the handle would flip the lock back closed! It did this over and over, and I didn't know what was happening. After yelling out to the people waiting in line just outside of the door, they tried to alert the owners of the stall. I waited a few minutes, tried again, and WHOOSH - the door opened! I do not fully know was going on there, but it scared me just enough to tell my family what had happened as soon as I got back to the concert area. This caused my grandmother, a former nurse, to say, "You sure have been going to the bathroom a lot today, how often are you getting up each night to use the restroom?" I thought about this quietly before saying, "Hmmm… probably six or seven?" My grandma figured it was diabetes, but she didn't want to worry us unnecessarily, so she suggested that I set an appointment with my doctor as soon as possible. A week later, when I went in for what I thought was a regular check-up, I was really worried that I would need to get an injection at this appointment. I hated needles, so the whole way there I remember asking my mom, "We're not getting a shot today, right Mom? We're just doing a check-up, they're not giving me any shots?" To which my mother of course replied that no, we were not going to the doctor for shots today. Little did we know that after that day I would have to have shots for the rest of my life.

When the doctor told me that I had diabetes, I did not believe her. This was uncharacteristic of me; I am usually an extremely trusting person and I had been going to this doctor for years, but when you get a diagnosis like that something in your brain switches to instant denial. I thought: *No, I don't have diabetes. Only old people get diabetes.* But my blood sugar was over 500 mg/dL, and we were on our way to the hospital to stay overnight. We were told that I could not even go home first to pack a bag. If you are a person with diabetes, you know what happens next: IVs, inpatient hospitalization, 24/7 monitoring, and a bombardment of information on your new diabetes diagnosis. It was all so overwhelming. My family and I knew absolutely nothing about diabetes, and I was terrified of needles. I cried at every single blood sugar check and insulin shot, and I did not want to learn how to do them for myself. After three days, I went home with a new diabetes kit and a hazy sense of the fact that my life had changed forever.

My biggest challenge was getting used to the needles. It took me over a year to fully come to terms with my diagnosis, and even longer than that to learn how to give my own shots. I went through various stages of denial, sadness, and wondering "Why me?" My endocrinologist suggested a therapist (who also happened to have Type 1 diabetes) who could help me with my fear of needles. The first step was just leaving needles in various places around the house, so I would get used to seeing them around. There were needles by the TV, in the bathroom, by the front door – anywhere in sight! Next I would draw up the insulin on my own, but still have my parents insert the needle, then eventually I would add pinching the skin up on my own, then pushing in the medicine on my own, and finally the last step – inserting the needle! For each milestone that I achieved I got a reward, such as a new toy or a fun trip. The day that I finally put a needle into my own body was a huge moment for me. There is just something about giving yourself a shot. You know you need the insulin and that you should just do it, but there is a mental block. Your brain tells you: *No! Don't hurt yourself!* And yet you know that you have to. It probably took me over a half hour after loading up the insulin syringe that day – but I finally put the needle in all by myself! My mom and I were jumping around the room at this major accomplishment.

From there, diabetes started to get easier. Was it still tons of work? Yes, that part has surely never changed, but it started to become more of a normal part of my life. My diabetes care began to become routine, automatic even! Along with this came a fascination with diabetes and its intricacies. Everything diabetes-related began to interest me greatly, and from there grew a desire to become a Certified Diabetes Educator, and to use all that I have learned about this disease to help others with the same diagnosis. Today, I use an insulin pump and a continuous glucose monitor, my A1C is the lowest it has ever been, and I have fully accepted my diabetes diagnosis. Are there still hard days? Sure, and there always will be because that comes with the unpredictability of this disease and its fluctuating blood sugars. But, each day I choose not to dwell on the negatives, and instead continue to do everything that I have always dreamed of, with my diabetes as just another part of this crazy journey.

Question 3: What are your top 3 tips for thriving with diabetes that you believe have served you (and continue to serve you) best along your diabetes journey?

1. Take it one day (maybe sometimes even one blood sugar) at a time.

2. Choose happiness.

3. Don't let diabetes stop you.

First, take it one day at a time. When you think about the big picture and how you are going to be doing all of this work for your diabetes for the rest of your life, it can seem pretty daunting. That is why I prefer not to think of it that way. Of course, you need to have some sense of the big picture in order to notice trends in your blood sugar and plan ahead. However, overall, I try to just focus on here and now. If I focus on making *today's* blood sugars good, and doing the best that I can right now, eventually all of those blood sugars will add up to an A1C that I can be proud of at my next endocrinologist appointment. When you break it into these manageable chunks of time, it seems much more do-able.

Second, choose happiness. Happiness is a choice. Done. End of story. If you let your happiness rest on your circumstances, you are never going to be happy. Life will never be perfect, and things will always go wrong, so it is up to you to make the best of it! Sometimes it is perfectly valid to have negative, sad, even angry feelings, but you cannot let them fester. I had a mourning period after I was diagnosed where I mourned the loss of my old "normal" life and had to accept my new one, but after that I needed to get on with the rest of my life! Take that time to be sad, but then turn it around and use it to grow and move forward. Diabetes is full of ups and downs in blood sugars, which can lead to ups and downs in our moods, but when I'm having a bad diabetes day (or a bad day in general) I find that I really can choose to be happy in spite of it. Blood sugars fluctuate; they just do. So try not to beat yourself up about every little out of range number, and instead just do what you can to fix it. After that, make a conscious effort to focus on the good in your day (or life!) and you will be much happier. It has always worked for me!

Thirdly, do not let diabetes stop you! For the most part, anything a non-diabetic can do, I can do too. I just need to put more work into it to make sure that I am prepared, and in the best possible control of my blood sugars. I have a couple of extra steps, a couple of extra tasks to help me complete my goals, but I still pursue them! I played sports all through high school, have gotten two college degrees, made it through an accelerated nursing program, have travelled overseas by myself by plane, done road trips by car, and studied abroad for months at a time. I live my life, and diabetes comes along, but I can handle it. I have been doing this for a while now and there are many others doing it too. I will not let it stop me.

Question 4: Is there anything else you would like to share that you think will add value to the readers?

I would like to say that another thing that has helped me in this crazy diabetes experience of mine is support from others. There is just something about meeting another person with diabetes that makes you feel better. I always joke that when I meet a new person with diabetes, I am thinking, "You are now my new best friend", but there is some truth beneath that humor. Other diabetics just understand certain aspects of your life that most non-diabetics never will. You can make diabetes jokes that most people would NEVER get the reference for, and you do not have to filter out certain aspects of your life from people who simply will not understand the lingo, or even the context. So, if you have not done so yet, I would encourage all people with diabetes to reach out. Go to a diabetes camp, conference, seminar, support group, or online community. Find others that you click with, and learn from each other! And for those non-diabetics in your life, try opening up a little more to them too. Try explaining diabetes to your close friends and you will see how quickly they catch on! I have numerous close friends who I have known and been open with for so long that they truly "get" this whole diabetes thing. When they ask how I am, I can mention diabetes without having to filter or explain, and that is pretty special. The people in your life are so important in this journey.

Subscribe to Danica on *YouTube:*

https://www.youtube.com/user/DiabeticDanica

EDWARD FIEDER

Question 1: Who are you? What makes you happy? What hobbies are you passionate about? Who do you love? What do you do for a living? Essentially, your bio plus some personal stuff!

Wait…You don't know who I am? Well allow ME to fill the void in YOUR life. My name is Edward Fieder and I am the creator of the Faces of Diabetes where we help change the way people view diabetes.

I am a photographer and re-toucher living in Alabama, and photography and videography are my main two loves. I enjoy making photos of things and situations that can't exist in real life, and I enjoy making videos that make fun of situations that do exist in real life. There's comedy in everything, and I like to think that I help bring it out. I love my family, friends, and people who support the Faces of Diabetes. Without their support the Faces of Diabetes wouldn't exist. I also, in no particular order, love kit kats, dogs, 50mm 1.4 camera lens, Disney, Coke Zero, books, diabetes, embarrassing squirrels, putt putt, hammocks, sleeping when it's raining, sleeping when it's not raining, crying openly to the Little Mermaid, sleeping, softboxes, not running marathons, my pump, Xbox, treasure, and sneezing.

Question 2: What is your diabetes story? Please share your story of diagnosis and the path you traveled to get where you are today. What have been your biggest struggles/triumphs in regard to living with diabetes? How does diabetes makes you awesome at life? What are the tools you use to manage your diabetes day to day (pump, MDI, CGM, etc.)?

My diabetes story CAN'T be told in less than 2,000 words. I can talk about my story for DAYS. Here's the shorter version. I was diagnosed at 11 and it was a tough pill to swallow. I had seen what diabetes could do to someone, and I thought that was what I had to look forward to. I became rebellious in my later teenage years with my diabetes care, but thankfully that passed before anything awful happened. I didn't know of many people with diabetes in the city I lived in, and I always felt like I was alone. I always wanted a diabetic best friend who could relate to all things diabetes, but it never happened. I think that's why I always felt at home at diabetes camp and encourage everyone young and old to get involved with their nearest one. I was both a camper and a counselor at a diabetes camp for a few years, and now do a lot of their media work. Jumping around, I graduated high school and went to college with no diabetes issues. I majored in graphic design and photography, and before I could graduate I had to do an exhibit show on a topic of my choosing. I was encouraged to do "living with diabetes" as my topic, but rejected the idea because I didn't want people to think that's all I was about. I played the diabetes card up a lot in school and now was my time to show people that there was more to me than JUST diabetes. Well…three rejected ideas later and the deadline was closing in… sooooo living with diabetes it was! The exhibit consisted of 7 images and a video depicting what my life had been like growing up with diabetes. Each one had a different reason/story behind it and it took me 4 months to complete. I made an A, graduated, and moved out to Colorado. While I was there I wanted to keep the exhibit going but I was out of ideas. My story had been told and I didn't know what else to do. That's when my dad came up with the idea that I should create a photo book filled with photos of people who live with diabetes. I am a photographer after all, and thus the Faces of Diabetes was born! Of course, it's grown into a lot more than JUST a photo book now. We now focus not only on the book, we also feature others' stories on our website and various social media accounts, and create comedic videos depicting some common and uncommon diabetes related incidents. Go check out the project yourself and you'll see why diabetes not only makes me awesome at life, but also so many others whose faces are waiting to be seen and voices ready to be heard! I hope the Faces of Diabetes inspires and encourages people to thrive with their diabetes instead of being depressed or upset about it. There's enough grief involved with diabetes...we are going to change that!

Oh yea...I'm on a Medtronic pump and Novalog. That's what's up!

Question 3: What are your top 3 tips for thriving with diabetes that you believe have served you (and continue to serve you) best along your diabetes journey?

Top 3 tips!

1.) EXERCISE!!! Just do it...go for a walk, ride a bike, jazzercise, juggle watermelons....WHATEVER it takes to get you moving for at least 30 minutes a day...GET IT DONE. It will do wonders for your diabetes management. BUT whatever you do...DO NOT exercise when your blood sugar is too high or low!

2.) Get into the habit of checking your blood sugar regularly. It may take a few days or weeks to get the hang of it but it's so important. It LITERALLY takes 5 seconds to get your number. Meters in the past took over 5 minutes...it's such a luxury now! If it's high then try and fix it...if it's low...then EAT! Also, make a couple extra diabetes-readiness packs and put one in your car, purse, backpack, etc so you are always ready to treat any lows. And if you have extra glucose meters laying around like many of us do, put those in the packs too, that way you never have an excuse for NOT checking your blood sugar no matter where you are.

3.) Get involved with the diabetes community, whether in person or online. Whether it be ADA, JDRF, a diabetes camp or support group, GET INVOLVED! Being associated with like-minded people and getting together and being awesome will work wonders on how you feel about this disease.

Question 4: Is there anything else you would like to share that you think will add value to the readers?

Keep up the good fight and treat your body right. Treatments are getting better...soon it'll be almost like we don't have diabetes at all! Just have to hold on and be patient!

I also love mail, surprises, insulin, breathing, Hey Arnold, Photoshop, 407, Harry Potter, making up statistics, VGHS but just the first season, Wacom, perfect blood sugars, diabetes camps, go karts, when the printer works without me having to get up and punch it, pizza, pirates, music, hot showers, beating Mario Bros., fall and winter in Alabama, Daniele Hargenrader, not being dead, taming stallions, night time, grooming my beard, throwing rocks at non-diabetics...just kidding...but seriously.

thefacesofdiabetes.org

RIVA GREENBERG

Question 1: Who are you? What makes you happy? What hobbies are you passionate about? Who do you love? What do you do for a living? Essentially, your bio plus some personal stuff!

My name is Riva Greenberg. I live in Brooklyn where I was actually born, although my parents moved two weeks later. Ah, the prodigal daughter returns. Travel seems to be a thread in my life and that suits me perfectly. When I was in college, I spent a semester studying abroad in Copenhagen, and training across Europe. When I was thirty-two, I moved to Tokyo and lived and worked there for a Japanese ad agency for six years. While in Japan, I traveled across Asia and Pan Asia. I have never wanted that international door to close, and it seems having married a man who grew up in Holland it never will.

But for now, Brooklyn suits me right down to the ground. Urban neighborhoods filled with charming brownstones, and leafy streets with Manhattan a stone's throw away. This actually Dutch, Indonesian guy who asked me to marry him fourteen years ago and I, live in a typically small city apartment. The fact that we haven't gotten divorced must mean we have a very good marriage.

Actually we do, and on top of it all we sometimes work together; he partners with me on some of my diabetes projects. He's an academic, an executive advisor, and he facilitates executive leadership workshops. He's also a thought leader and an expert on sustainable performance improvement. In short, we are combining silos; bringing his management expertise to diabetes management. It is an innovative thing to do in healthcare where silos rarely if ever cross. And, it is breeding results in how to live more positively with diabetes.

Daniele talks about creating a life in which you thrive with diabetes, and that is exactly what we are working on. Specifically, a treatment approach for health professionals, and a mindset for people living with diabetes, that we call the Flourishing Approach. I began my work in diabetes interviewing more than 150 people who live with it. I saw many were living a thriving life. I realized early on in this work, you can have a great life not *despite*, but *because* of diabetes. For many people, diabetes is just the wake up call they need to get healthier, and find their purpose in life.

My greatest joy is sharing with others who have diabetes and health professionals what I know about living a healthy, happy life with diabetes. I love seeing the light go on in someone's eyes when they see new possibilities for themselves. My friends would also say I love good food, great wine, soul-searching conversations, movies, books, travel, and living in a world of possibilities.

Question 2: What is your diabetes story? Please share your story of diagnosis and the path you traveled to get where you are today. What have been your biggest struggles/triumphs in regard to living with diabetes? How does diabetes makes you awesome at life? What are the tools you use to manage your diabetes day to day (pump, MDI, CGM, etc.)?

I woke in my parent's house screaming in pain. I was having the same excruciating leg cramps I'd been having for almost three months. Home, on a winter break from college, my parents and I bundled into the car for what we thought would be a routine doctor visit. A few simple blood tests later, I was told I had a blood sugar level of 750 and juvenile diabetes, now known as type 1 diabetes.

I was 18 then. I was put in the hospital for four days. I remember the tape loop in my head, "Why me?" I also remember the woman in the bed next to me who had numbers tattooed on her arm. She was a survivor of the Holocaust. I remember how when she was in pain and the nurses didn't come, I would run down the hall to get medication for her. One thing I know about myself is that I have always had a keen sense of justice, and will always fight for the underdog.

When I got out of the hospital, my diabetes faded into the background of my life. It was 1972. There would be no glucose meters until 1982. I took one shot of insulin in the morning, and was told not to eat candy bars. As more information came out through the years, I learned about food, diet, exercise, stress, and medicine. I got better at managing my diabetes with these tools. But it was at a TCOYD conference when psychologist/CDE Bill Polonsky uttered words that would elevate my diabetes management. He said, "Diabetes does not cause blindness, heart attacks, kidney disease and amputation. Poorly managed diabetes does."

After hearing those words, I had an entirely new sense that I could truly influence my health with my actions. I have lived that way ever since, and it has paid off. After 43 years with Type 1 diabetes, I have no complications.

My personal interest in diabetes has always been on the emotional side. The thing we talk least about: how do you get up each and every day and stay resilient managing this disease?

Personally, in my twenties and thirties I didn't share my diabetes with anyone. I didn't want diabetes to be the center of attention, and I thought, who could understand the micromanagement Type 1 diabetes demands? Why would I burden anyone with this? So, my diabetes sat there with me and with my friends, me and a date, but stayed quiet. I didn't even know anyone with diabetes during that time. Then, when I turned 40, for some reason I really don't recall, I shared it with everyone, and well, it hasn't stopped.

When I was forty-eight years old, I had a true turning point that led me to work in diabetes as a patient expert. I was planning my wedding, my *first* thank you, seeing a diabetes educator for the first time after thirty- two years with diabetes, and going into the hospital for frozen shoulder surgery. I had also just lost my job.

Looking for a new position, and thinking after seeing the diabetes educator I'd like to help people with diabetes, my husband suggested I write a book about what it's like to live with diabetes. I looked at him sweetly, rolled my eyes and said, "Honey, who's going to buy a book about what I *think* about living with diabetes?!" Since then, I've written three books and hundreds of articles, and speak onstage and off at international and national health conferences. There's something to be said for putting your dreams out there.

I am lucky. I don't find it unnecessarily burdensome to take care of my diabetes. I eat very similarly day to day, a low carb diet. I've grown to love my flax seed muffins and roasted vegetables, and don't feel I'm sacrificing as bagel-lovers will accuse me of. My taste buds love the taste of nourishing wholesome foods, and so does my blood sugar which stays in range on my low carb regimen.

I walk every morning for an hour, and have just started weight training. People always ask me if I wear a pump, and the answer is no. I take multiple injections. I'm so used to them that I don't really mind, and I don't want the weight of a pump on my body. I do have a CGM, and use it but not every day. Since my days are so routine and I work at home and can control my environment, I usually wear the CGM when I'm traveling and everything goes topsy turvy.

Personally, I see diabetes as my teacher. It has shown me how strong and capable I am. It reminds me how fortunate I am that what I have is manageable, especially as many of my peers are now leaving the world too soon. Diabetes has made me a little more fearless than I would have been without it. It has led me to work I love, and amazing people who share this work with me. I don't know if one is optimistic by nature or nurture, but I am optimistic – about my present and my future. So much so that I've already applied for my Joslin 50 year medal while still seven and a half years away!

In the words of Mahatma Gandhi, "Happiness is when what you think, what you say, and what you do are in harmony." I'm pretty happy.

Question 3: What are your top 3 tips for thriving with diabetes that you believe have served you (and continue to serve you) best along your diabetes journey?

1. <u>Routine</u> – We seldom talk about it, but doing mostly the same things routinely each day makes your blood sugars easier to manage, because it's a lot more predictable. I know there are people for whom eating the same meal two days in a row would be a travesty, but not for me. Eat similarly, exercise similarly, and you'll notice how much easier diabetes becomes to manage.

2. <u>Learn everything you can</u> – Oprah said it, "The more you know, the better you do." I tell people this all the time. You may spend a handful of hours a year with your health care providers. That leaves over 8, 860 hours a year that you're on your own. Besides, whose diabetes is it? Learn everything you can – read books, magazines, articles, take a class, join a support group, start chatting on social media web sites. Learn so much that you can't help but find yourself sharing with others how much you know.

3. <u>Diabetes friends</u> – It's so hard to realize I didn't know anyone with diabetes my first twenty years living with the disease. Today, I probably have more friends who *have* diabetes than who don't. There's nothing like the "I get it" factor that warms the heart when it comes to living with this disease. Whether you're confused, blue, happy, ecstatic, fearful, anything, sharing it with a diabetes friend is like picking the frosted roses off the cake – sweet. Yes pun intended. There's an amazing bond among people with diabetes, always a ready hand extended, and it can soothe or set your soul soaring.

Question 4: Is there anything else you would like to share that you think will add value to the readers?

My mantra last year was "Be bold." My mantra this year is "Be bolder." Go after your dreams, do your best, why else are we here? One of my favorite quotes is, "Be brave with your life so that others can be brave with theirs." It is not about ego; it is not egotistical to let your light shine. It is a beacon you are holding for others to help them live their best life.

You can find Riva's books online:

Diabetes Do's & How-To's

50 Diabetes Myths That Can Ruin Your Life and the 50 Diabetes Truths That Can Save It

The ABCs Of Loving Yourself With Diabetes

DiabetesStories.com

DiabetesbyDesign.com

Huffington Post

Daniele Hargenrader

SHAYLYN LEAHY

Question 1: Who are you? What makes you happy? What hobbies are you passionate about? Who do you love? What do you do for a living? Essentially, your bio plus some personal stuff!

My name is Shaylyn Leahy; I'm 21 years old and currently a full time student at Bloomsburg University. I am a nursing major, and will soon be starting my senior year. In addition to being a full time student, I work as a certified nursing assistant (CNA) in a pediatric cardiac intensive care unit at St. Christopher's hospital. Things that make me happy are my friends, my family, my dog, exercising, summer, and the beach! I spend my free time reading, studying, watching TV, cooking, exercising and hanging out with my friends and family. I love my dog more than life and my friends and family mean the world to me.

Question 2: What is your diabetes story? Please share your story of diagnosis and the path you traveled to get where you are today. What have been your biggest struggles/triumphs in regard to living with diabetes? How does diabetes makes you awesome at life? What are the tools you use to manage your diabetes day to day (pump, MDI, CGM, etc.)?

I was diagnosed with diabetes when I was ten years old. I went in for my annual physical and was asked to give a urine sample, which my doctors found contained glucose. They immediately sent me to the hospital. When I was first diagnosed I had never even heard of diabetes and thought I was going to die, then while in the hospital I learned that diabetes wasn't as bad as I thought. For about a year after I was diagnosed I managed my diabetes with insulin injections, and eventually my parents and doctors agreed that I would be able to use a pump. From then on I used an insulin pump, which has made

275

my life so much easier. I was in middle school when I first got the pump and it made such a difference in my self-esteem, being able to go over my friends' houses and not carry a bag of needles and insulin. I didn't really struggle with diabetes until my freshman year of high school, when I began to rebel. I didn't want to have diabetes anymore, I stopped caring about what I ate and would just eat food regardless of what it would do to my blood sugar. My A1c went up and I was going through what many individuals refer to as "Diabetes Burnout." The poor control of my diabetes was a big stressor in my relationship with my parents. I did not want to hear what they had to say, and would constantly fight with them about it. Eventually around my junior year of high school my mom had had enough. She had taken me to counseling, and even tried scare tactics by telling me horror stories of people getting their limbs amputated hoping that would get me to want to take better care of my diabetes. My mom found an article in the local newspaper about a trainer who had diabetes, and who had struggled with her diabetes as well, and that trainer was Daniele. Reluctantly, I agreed to meet with her, and it ended up being one of the greatest things for my relationship with diabetes. I have been working with Daniele ever since and I have had many ups and downs with my diabetes over the years. I began exercising more and realized how amazing I actually feel when I exercise and eat right. My biggest struggle with diabetes has been trying to learn not to beat myself up about having a high blood sugar or not always eating healthy food. I continue to struggle with this obstacle even to this day, but I do the best that I can every day. I still learn every day about how my body reacts to new experiences, and foods I haven't tried before. I recently began using a CGM along with my pump, and it has been so useful in seeing how my blood sugar reacts to everything at the push of a button. Although having diabetes has been a struggle at times, I don't think I would be the person I am today without it. As crazy as that sounds, having diabetes has helped me pick my nursing career, made me a stronger person, and has taught me so many life lessons. I truly believe that if

I did not have diabetes I would not be as interested in eating healthy and exercising as I am today.

Question 3: What are your top 3 tips for thriving with diabetes that you believe have served you (and continue to serve you) best along your diabetes journey?

1) Exercise consistently, it makes you feel great!
2) Eat healthy most of the time, but don't feel guilty having a treat every now and then.
3) Don't be so hard on yourself. Do the best that you can do at any given moment. Learn from your mistakes and move on. Don't dwell on them or beat yourself up about it.

Question 4: Is there anything else you would like to share that you think will add value to the readers? Diabetes sucks sometimes, but remember we are more than this disease! We control our choices when it comes to our diabetes, they do not control you!

Twitter: @shaybaybay628

MAUREEN "REENIE" MONTGOMERY

Question 1: Who are you? What makes you happy? What hobbies are you passionate about? Who do you love? What do you do for a living? Essentially, your bio plus some personal stuff!

My name is Maureen Montgomery, but I go by Reenie. I am 48 years young and I live in Iowa. Making others smile and helping people makes me happy. I also enjoy painting, reading, gardening, camping and watching movies. I love the water, and that includes boating, swimming, canoeing...pretty much anything involving water! It's my peaceful place. I am a 911 Dispatcher. I really enjoy my work, but it can be extremely stressful at times! My family, friends, and coworkers help me to de-stress. They are my rocks!

Question 2: What is your diabetes story? Please share your story of diagnosis and the path you traveled to get where you are today. What have been your biggest struggles/triumphs in regard to living with diabetes? How does diabetes makes you awesome at life? What are the tools you use to manage your diabetes day to day (pump, MDI, CGM, etc.)?

I have type 2 diabetes, and I was diagnosed in October of 2003. I have a huge family history of diabetes, so I felt like I was destined to have it eventually. I started with just diet and exercise for the first 8 years. Then, I moved to Metformin, and then to Kombiglyze. I began using Lantus insulin in February 2015. The biggest struggles for me have been odd work hours, and I love sweets. I have had my ups and downs throughout the years, including several burnout times. I have had the "Why me?" moments as well. I have not had a lot of family support, as my immediate family lives in Texas and I live in Iowa. Previously, I was married to someone who was in denial about my diabetes. I am now divorced from him. I did most of my diabetes management on my own for a long time. I struggled with making healthy meals when my ex-husband wanted things with carbs that were not healthy for me. I kept my diabetes a secret from most of my friends and coworkers, because I was embarrassed. After divorcing, I have finally accepted my diabetes, and am doing much better. In September, 2011, I joined the website DLife and met a friend on there who I opened up to. He is also a type 2, and we bonded almost immediately. He lives in another state, and we are still friends today. With his encouragement and support, I started to tell a few coworkers and friends about my diabetes. Now everyone I work with knows I have diabetes, and I am no longer embarrassed. I have now met a wonderful man, who I am now engaged to (update, they've gotten married!), who enjoys helping me make better eating choices. We exercise together, and I have hopes for a very bright future!

Question 3: What are your top 3 tips for thriving with diabetes that you believe have served you (and continue to serve you) best along your diabetes journey?

- Eat healthy as often as you can. I have found a low carb diet works best for me!

- Find websites about diabetes that can give you all the information you can find, as well as great recipes! Maybe you can find a friend on there too!

- Exercise as often as you can. Daily or every other day works best for me!

- You are going to have days where you "fall off the wagon". Try not to beat yourself up about it. Just jump back on the wagon the next day! You can do this!

Question 4: Is there anything else you would like to share that you think will add value to the readers?

For me, it helps knowing there are others like me that sometimes struggle with diabetes management and staying on track. I feel like I am part of a team, and we work together. If I can help one person with this, I am a happy camper! Find what makes YOU happy, and do more of that! Good luck, and stay strong and healthy!

STEPHEN NULTY

Question 1: Who are you? What makes you happy? What hobbies are you passionate about? Who do you love? What do you do for a living? Essentially, your bio plus some personal stuff!

First of all I would like to say a big "thank you" to Daniele for asking me to contribute to her book. My name is Stephen Nulty and I have been living with diabetes since 1987. Later you will find out all about my challenges and success, but in the meanwhile, let me give you a bit of background on me.

From a young age I have been a massive fan of football (soccer for Americans!) As a result of this I focused all my energy and spare time on playing as much football as I could. It was my life, my purpose, and my dream. Fortunately I was able to fulfill the dream of being paid to play football in my mid-twenties by playing for a team in Iceland called Huggin on the east coast. I was also fortunate to play at college level in the States for Piedmont College in Demorest, GA. Despite my love for football, I soon turned to property around 2002 and starting investing in new builds and buying single lets to build a property portfolio which I still have to this day. As you can imagine diabetes is also a big part of my life, and around 2014 I set up a website called Diabetes Mastery with the aim to support and help other people with diabetes around the world learn more about living with diabetes and how diet can have a profound effect if taking seriously.

My hobbies vary from football as you know, to snowboarding, and recently I've taken up sailing. Whoever tells you that diabetes is going to stop you from doing things is either ignorant or uneducated. Diabetes IS manageable and should not affect your goals in life. For me, it was a spring board to my achievements.

Question 2: What is your diabetes story? Please share your story of diagnosis and the path you traveled to get where you are today. What have been your biggest struggles/triumphs in regard to living with diabetes? How does diabetes makes you awesome at life? What are the tools you use to manage your diabetes day to day (pump, MDI, CGM, etc.)?

In 1987 after visiting the optician and being prescribed glasses, I started to frequent the toilet a lot more than usual. This increased over a 3 week period, and before I knew it I was extremely ill in bed sweating and drinking a lot of liquids, mainly sugary drinks. I couldn't hold it though and after several days of getting worse my mother called the doctor. He came out several times while I was ill and put it down to a virus before my mother, taking the initiative, called the hospital herself. She also informed the doctor who came out at the same time as the ambulance arrived and diagnosed me with appendicitis. While on my way to the hospital the paramedics did all the usual tests and discovered that I did in fact have diabetes. My sugar levels where reading "Hi" as their monitoring devices could not give an actual reading. Whilst on the way to the hospital, I would then slip in to a coma and find myself in hospital for the next 6 weeks. The coma only lasted approximately 24 hours, however, I do recall waking up extremely thirsty and attached to a drip. I was 10 years old.

The doctors would wait until I was in better health before informing me that I had diabetes. I remember looking at them and saying, "Ok, can I go play football now?" I had no idea what diabetes was, nor could I even think about the implications it would have on my life. I recall my parents being more upset about it than I was. I guess even back then I had a very positive attitude towards life. From then on in I treated every day as a bonus. And why not, earlier I was in a coma and technically I should have died if it were not for the medical staff at the hospital, Dr. Frederick Banting and student Charles Best (Dr. Banting and his student Charles Best are the guys that discovered insulin in 1920).

I was so grateful to be alive, and for all the help I received. I promised myself I would not let my life go to waste.

The next 20 years of my life would be a time of learning from the "medical experts" and managing my diabetes with varying results. The early years were very good for me, however in my late twenties I was starting to struggle with control and found it extremely difficult to maintain good sugar levels. It was affecting my work day, and most importantly my football. I visited the doctor often and would ask for help to get back on track. After a period of time I would start to see a pattern, and started to ask different questions of the medical industry. Questions like, "Is anyone of these doctors actually diabetic?", "Why is there a headline in the papers every 5 years saying the cure is in trials and only 5 years away?", "Why do I have diabetes?", "Is there a cure?" Now you might be thinking, why didn't you ask these questions earlier? I did, but only to myself. I had faith in the medical industry back then. I had hope!

In 2007 my life was turned upside down when I went to a course to learn about nutrition, detoxing, how the body actually works, and how an education in health could actually benefit me called *Life Mastery* put on by Tony Robbins. I turned up at the event and got extremely worried when they told me that as part of the detox I would receive no solid food. I was panicking and sought advice from one of the trainers. I'll never forget the conversation. I asked her, "What I should do?" She told me that she was no doctor, but asked why I take insulin. I told her to lower my blood sugar levels. She responded with, "You will not be getting any sugar this week, other than some from fruits." My jaw hit the floor, but it opened up a new mindset for me. I said *okay, lets experiment.* If I'm not getting any processed sugar, then I won't take any insulin! Please note that I am not advising any people with diabetes to not take their insulin. Also you should note that I was on Actrapid and Lantus back then, so I was taking a fast acting and a long acting insulin. I only stopped my fast acting insulin. I continued to take my long acting.

The results that week blew me away. I learned the value of nature's foods, salads, fruits, veg, nuts and seeds. The benefits of living foods and how they impact the body. You see, living foods such as green leafy vegetables are high in alkalinity which the supports the bodies PH levels. I was stunned at the results in just 6 days of eliminating processed sugar and living off juices made from fruit and veg. I was hooked, and would spend the next 2 years learning as much as I could about my body, my diet, and how to get optimal health. It has been a rollercoaster ever since with many more ups than downs. I came home after the event and immediately turned to a raw food lifestyle after spending my entire life up until that point eating meat, fried foods, and anything else processed you can think of. Within days I had reduced my fast acting insulin from 10 units per meal to 3 or 4. My long acting insulin was reduced from 20 to 12 units and my overall health was amazing. I had a color in my face never before seen and my energy increased tenfold.

These days I mix it up and eat both raw and cooked foods, although I have not touched milk or meat since 2007. I will eat the occasional egg and have the occasional fish. Other than that I am still learning about my body and always changing as I grow older. For me, there is not one way of eating that fits all. It is always about calibration and adjusting to life's demands and your lifestyle.

Today I use the Humalog pen for fast acting insulin and Lantus for my long acting. I'm currently on 6/12 units of Humalog per meal and 15 units of Lantus. My weight is stable, and twice a year I do a detox of my own to cleanse my system and reset myself at a cellular level. I monitor my blood sugar levels before each meal and also before and after exercise.

Question 3: What are your top 3 tips for thriving with diabetes that you believe have served you (and continue to serve you) best along your diabetes journey?

Accountability, responsibility and ownership. These are my top 3 tips. It wasn't until I took ownership of my diabetes that I could then take responsibility and accountability for my actions. I am the one living with it, not my doctors or family. For too long I was looking for answers outside of myself. We live in a world where 70% of the world's knowledge is accessible via a computer. We have more experts than ever before. The days of not knowing or not seeking help are gone. We no longer can blame others for our management habits. When I was first diagnosed, there were 200,000 children in the UK with type 1 diabetes. Very few people knew what it was or how to deal with it. We were all learning together. The world is now in a pandemic with over 350 million people with diabetes. To this day I accept that it is my choice regarding how I manage my diabetes. Don't get me wrong, its tiring, it's frustrating, it's a pain in the ass at times, but it's the hand I was dealt and there is none better to deal with it than me. I know how I feel after eating certain foods, I know how I feel after exercise therefore I can do something about it. My advice to any persona with diabetes is to take it seriously, and educate yourself on what works and what doesn't work for you and make the changes you need to feel your best.

diabetesmastery.com

GABRIELLE SHARKEY-OLDFIELD

Question 1: Who are you? What makes you happy? What hobbies are you passionate about? Who do you love? What do you do for a living? Essentially, your bio plus some personal stuff!

My name is Gabrielle Sharkey Oldfield; I'm 49 years old, and I am a full-time pastor and a part-time sales engineer. I am married to my wonderful husband, Bob, and between us we have four great kids ages 18-24. I am happiest when I'm outside hiking, kayaking, or snowshoeing. I love to challenge myself to go longer or farther, and I love to encourage people to come along with me. I enjoy cooking, read when I can, and have recently started running 5ks. I'm not fast, but it is so fun to see my stats slowly get better over time.

Question 2: What is your diabetes story? Please share your story of diagnosis and the path you traveled to get where you are today. What have been your biggest struggles/triumphs in regard to living with diabetes? How does diabetes makes you awesome at life? What are the tools you use to manage your diabetes day to day (pump, MDI, CGM, etc.)?

I was diagnosed with Type 1 diabetes less than a year ago in December 2014, at 48 years of age. Over the previous two years, I had been working on losing weight and getting healthier through outdoor activities, and trying to eat better without dieting. I was having great success and feeling amazing until late October/November of 2014. It was at that time I began to lose weight no matter what I ate or did. I lost energy, and had unquenchable thirst. One early morning I woke up and could not catch my breath, I didn't have the strength to walk, so my husband carried me to the car and prayed while rushing me to the ER that they would be able to figure out what was going on. Those prayers were answered when it took under a minute for the ER doctor to diagnose DKA and start treatment immediately. My blood sugar at that time was 590. I spent a few days in the ICU discovering that my entire life was about to change. I was blessed to have two amazing nurses during that time. One of those women showed me the compassion I needed to make it through the day, while the other was more down to business and made sure I knew how to inject basal and rapid acting insulin by myself (even when I didn't feel like practicing), while quizzing me on the signs of hypoglycemia. I am so very thankful for them both. I was released from the hospital and sent home, still reeling from all that had happened. Given my previous weight issues, I was sure the type 1 diagnosis was a mistake, but it wasn't.

My biggest struggle in the beginning (and sometimes even now) is getting information I can actually use. I was terrified over those first couple of months. My vision was blurry; I didn't understand fully what the insulin did, and when I was told to eat X amount of carbs per meal and inject X amount of insulin—I did. I had terrible lows trying to follow this plan with no knowledge of how or if I could make my own adjustments.

I went online and found a book called, "Think Like a Pancreas." It saved my life. Understanding that there was an actual relationship between all the factors in play at any given moment—carbs, food, emotions, exercise--and the resulting low or high blood sugars—gave me hope. Understanding that sometimes, even if I did everything right, I may get a result I didn't expect, helped free me from feeling like a failure. I bought an excellent app to track my blood sugar (MySugr), and immediately reaped benefits from seeing, with my own eyes, the results of certain foods, walking on the treadmill, or forgetting to bolus. It also gave me a great starting point when I was finally able to see an endocrinologist three weeks later.

I am only in my first year of diagnosis, and certainly still in my honeymoon phase, but going from an A1c of 10.9 to a 5.6 makes me feel a little less at the mercy of the insulin I need to survive. I joined a group that does strength training in rotating six week stints after reading about the positive effects of increased muscle and insulin sensitivity. I thought it would be a chore, but I love it, and the results have been outstanding and consistent. It gave me the incentive to try a Barre class that meets in the interim, and now that is a regular part of my life as well.

I never ran before, but I run now. I've made the joke that after the age of 8, I never ran for fun or on purpose, and that is pretty much the straight truth. There was something, however, about being told that I might want to be careful about taxing physical activities like running, which made me want to run. So, that being the case, I would say my biggest triumphs include that I have completed three 5ks so far this year, and am about to do number four. I did my first Mudderella obstacle course event (five miles, 12 obstacles) this year, and am still hiking, kayaking, and snowshoeing. I am seriously in the best shape I have ever been.

Diabetes has given me a greater compassion and empathy for those that struggle with any physical and medical afflictions. I want to be an encourager, a cheerleader, an example of what someone can do— because who doesn't want to feel better?

Currently the tools I use are my glucometer and syringes. I test, test, and test some more. Being able to make the connection between what is going on that day, my blood sugar numbers, and how I feel is powerful information. Seeing how exercise increases my insulin sensitivity helps keep me motivated. I may move to a pump at some point, but right now I am wielding my needles like a ninja.

I also consider reading and the internet both important tools. I want to know how to make my insulin work with the life I want to live, feel the best that I can feel, and have the least amount of complications possible. There is a wealth of information out there; I just make sure to do additional research to check the credibility and reliability of those resources.

Question 3: What are your top 3 tips for thriving with diabetes that you believe have served you (and continue to serve you) best along your diabetes journey?

Understand that what works for you might be different than what works for someone else. I read a lot, use what pertains to me, and tuck the rest away in case it becomes useful later.

Be realistic about your goals. Make them meaningful but not impossible. As you start hitting them, you will WANT to challenge yourself to see if you can bump it up a little. It is so rewarding to be able to see progress—no matter how big or small.

Put yourself out there so you can find support from other people with this disease, and so that you can BE that support as well. My learning curve has been greatly improved by my ability to talk to other people with diabetes. There have been many things I didn't have to learn the hard way because someone else did.

Question 4: Is there anything else you would like to share that you think will add value to the reader?

Don't be afraid. The first month after my diagnosis, everything I read seemed to start with a statistic about amputations, blindness, and nerve damage. Almost every person I talked to had some horrible story about someone they knew that had died from complications of diabetes. I was certain my life was over, and I cried a lot. Don't give that fear the time of day. You can do whatever it takes to feel good, and be happy and healthy. You are smart enough to figure out what works best for you. Commit to working this disease like a boss, and then do it!

www.theunbolusedcookie.com / Twitter: @GabeOldfield

STEVE PONDER

Question 1: Who are you? What makes you happy? What hobbies are you passionate about? Who do you love? What do you do for a living? Essentially, your bio plus some personal stuff!

I'm Steve Ponder. My personal journey with type 1 diabetes began on March 1, 1966. It was called "juvenile diabetes" back then. The forces underlying the origin of my form of diabetes would not be discovered for another 15 years. The label "type 1 diabetes" would eventually be what best described my diabetes. But regardless of its name, I've taken doses of insulin (by syringe, pen or pump) over the past 50 years to stay alive. Being "in control" is another matter altogether.

Happiness is like the tides. Sometimes it swells while at other points it can seem to recede into the distance. I'm consistently rewarded by helping others grow and develop, whether as patients living with a chronic disease like diabetes, or more recently as a pediatric residency director helping to lift up new doctors aspiring to become pediatricians.

Earlier in my life, I had hobbies such as coin collecting, ham radio, chess, and tennis (I was competitive in the latter two). As I grew older, I took on more individual activities, primarily walking. It was a great way to get away from the urgencies of the day. It's a great stress relief too.

I chose to become a doctor because of my diabetes, but had no grand plan for what I would do with it. It wasn't until I volunteered to serve at a children's diabetes camp in Texas that I knew what I wanted to do with my professional (and to a large extent personal) life. In 1990, I became a board certified pediatric endocrinologist. The year before, I attained the certified diabetes educator (CDE) credential, and have maintained that status ever since. I'm the 3rd longest certified MD, CDE in the country. I'm quite proud of that. I also had the privilege to be the chair of the National Certification Board for Diabetes Educators (NCBDE), the organization which oversees the maintenance and promotion of the CDE credential. I now serve as the medical director of the diabetes camp which started it all in 1981; 35 years and going strong. The camp has impacted my life in more ways than I can count. For example, one of my adult children chose to become an RD and aspires to become a CDE, plus met her husband at camp. None of my children have diabetes, but they all understand it quite well and have been a source of inspiration to take the best care of myself in anticipation of the day I may have grandchildren.

I've conducted both basic and clinical research over my professional career, plus led many local, state and national boards and task forces on child advocacy, diabetes, and childhood obesity. I recently wrote the book Sugar Surfing, which describes a paradigm changing approach to diabetes self-management. I have been conducting workshops on this method across the US and in Europe for the past few years.

I love to teach, and help people grasp new concepts. I've been a television, radio, and medical columnist over the past 25 years as well. Teaching is what I do. But, the most rewarding aspect is to see or hear from those I teach when they apply what they've learned in their personal lives and/or professional practices.

Question 2: What is your diabetes story? Please share your story of diagnosis and the path you traveled to get where you are today. What have been your biggest struggles/triumphs in regard to living with diabetes? How does diabetes makes you awesome at life? What are the tools you use to manage your diabetes day to day (pump, MDI, CGM, etc.)?

I was diagnosed with diabetes when I was 9 years old. My comprehension of it was very limited then. Education was not provided to me in a way I could understand it. I was simply told what I needed to do, not why. It was what we call today a "paternalistic approach", in other words, just do as the doctor said. There was no flexibility in my regimen. It was a one size fits all approach day after day. I actually experienced few diabetes obstacles in my youth, largely because my diabetes could be fairly transparent to others outside the home, and even at school. I didn't take insulin outside home, we didn't check blood sugar in those days, and I rarely got very low since my blood sugars were mostly high all the time. Privately, I felt I would not live very long, but kept those thoughts mostly to myself. It was actually a childhood triumph when I made it to the year 2000 and I was still alive. During my youth, I assumed that would not happen.

Having three children and watching them all grow into productive adults has been only matched by my 30 years of marriage to my wife Patsy, who has saved me from desperately low blood sugar events until I was able to develop Sugar Surfing.

My greatest diabetes tool is my brain. It contains a wealth of experience, and is how I use my knowledge to make the best care choices I can. I'm not always right, but I'm smart enough to learn from my errors, which is a trait of champions I aim to maintain. In the last few years, I've developed a philosophy about life with diabetes that some might consider morbid. By my reckoning, I should have died almost 50 years ago. In fact, people still do die with type 1 diabetes in places where access to insulin is scarce or not possible. I see each day I wake up as a gift. And, as such, I choose not to spend my time complaining or worrying about having diabetes. I certainly respect it, but I don't fear it anymore. It's how I stay positive in my approach to all my daily self-care choices, which truly defines what others call "control".

I have used an insulin pump for 30 years, but the last few years I've realized through Sugar Surfing that how I take my insulin takes a back seat to the choices I make as to when and how much gets taken. I maintain a mid-5% A1C with multi-dose insulin therapy on or off a pump. I liken this to the choice a driver makes between a manual or automatic transmission. Both get the job done, and neither really makes a big difference in the quality of the ride. That's handled by the person behind the steering wheel.

My meter and CGM are like my compass and GPS, respectively. These are the tools that complement my knowledge and experience, and how I can maintain the level of diabetes control I enjoy. But, a low A1C is not my true reward. That comes from the feeling of normalcy that being in control provides, combined with the sense of dominance I now wield over a disease which for decades I allowed to dominate me. No more.

Question 3: What are your top 3 tips for thriving with diabetes that you believe have served you (and continue to serve you) best along your diabetes journey?

Striving for a normal life is my guiding principle to dominating diabetes. We could spend our lives feeling broken, but I choose a different path. Things don't always happen as planned. Often just the opposite. I accept chaos as part of life, and certainly part of diabetes. I embrace this, and am always aiming to be prepared for the unexpected. That anticipation has gotten me out of many tight jams over time. Finally, as a Sugar Surfer, I aim to manage the flux and drift in my blood sugars, and do this with passion and enthusiasm each day. I never tire of the challenge. For me, this is an easy attitude to have when I see every day as a gift from God. I refuse to waste my time worrying, feeling guilty or second guessing myself. Our time on Earth is relatively brief, and I intend to make the most of it while I can.

Question 4: Is there anything else you would like to share that you think will add value to the readers?

As I enter my 7th decade of life, I want to change the way we approach our diabetes self-care. It's time for a paradigm shift. Dynamic diabetes management (also known as Sugar Surfing) is that shift whose time has arrived. This rejects the supremacy of fixed insulin doses and ratios, the precise measurement of carbs, and the false perception of predictability of diabetes outcomes if only a prepared algorithm or sliding scale is followed. It will take years to change hearts and minds. This is my mission. I'm doing it by example, the only way I know how. As others embrace the method, the message spreads.

You can find Steve's book online:

Sugar Surfing

sugarsurfing.com

BOBBIE ROBERTSON

Question 1: Who are you? What makes you happy? What hobbies are you passionate about? Who do you love? What do you do for a living? Essentially, your bio plus some personal stuff!

My name is Bobbie Robertson and I'm from Fort Worth, Texas. I have 4 sons and one daughter, ranging in age from 24 - 40, as well as 1 grandson and 4 granddaughters who are all living on the West Coast. I have been a teacher/professor for the last 45 years, built 3 multimillion dollar companies, and now have a thriving coaching and consulting company as my "retirement job". I am an avid reader, love food, traveling, bowling, and the theatre.

Question 2: What is your diabetes story? Please share your story of diagnosis and the path you traveled to get where you are today. What have been your biggest struggles/triumphs in regard to living with diabetes? How does diabetes makes you awesome at life? What are the tools you use to manage your diabetes day to day (pump, MDI, CGM, etc.)?

About 15 years ago I was overweight, in my late 40's, and always sick. I went to the doctor thinking something was very wrong because everything I ate made me sick, I was always either sweating, vomiting, or so weak and shaky that I had to sit down. I was having difficulty working, always exhausted, miserable and had no idea what was wrong with me. I was always "starving", thirsty, and had the most absurd food cravings.

After 3 visits to the doctor and about $1000.00 worth of tests I was diagnosed with type 2 diabetes. The doctor immediately put me on insulin injections 3 times per day, as well as Metformin. But no matter how hard I tried to follow the diet he instructed me to follow I could not get my blood sugar under control. It was all over the place and I was feeling even worse than when I started. After 10 years my A1c was still hovering at approximately 9.6.

I began to struggle with diabetic nerve pain in my feet and lower legs, the smallest wounds would not heal for weeks or even months. My hair began to fall out, my skin became so dry and flaky it was embarrassing, and my weight was a lost cause.

Then I met a doctor who specialized in non-traditional methods of treating diabetes. I thought he was a little bit of a quack, but by this time I was desperate enough to try anything. He made me throw out the traditional diabetes diet and replace it with a vegetarian / low carb diet. For 3 months, I was not allowed any meat, poultry, or fish, and my plate was required to be 2/3 green vegetables. My carbs were limited to one serving per meal and I had to walk 3 times per week for at least 30 minutes. At the end of 3 months my A1c was down to 7.2.

Then, he encouraged me to give up diet sodas, walk 5 times per week, add 2 liters of water per day and begin to drink a green juice once a day that consisted of 6 lbs. of pressed kale in every 12 ounce bottle. I must admit, it was the nastiest stuff I had ever put in my mouth and made me gag every time I drank it, but by the end of the second 3 months my A1C was at 5.8. Talk about a drastic difference in my quality of health and the quality of my day to day life!

The effort was worth it! I lost 125 lbs., brought my A1c from 9.6 to 5.8 in 6 months, and for the first time in over 10 years I actually felt good. I stopped taking all insulin and now only take Metformin once per day. Life is really good right now. I have more strength, better health, and more energy than I have had in 40 years. And yes, I still drink the nasty stuff every day. It is a small price to pay for feeling good!

Question 3: What are your top 3 tips for thriving with diabetes that you believe have served you (and continue to serve you) best along your diabetes journey?

1. Eat a lot more green vegetables.

2. Exercise more.

3. Drink more water.

Question 4: Is there anything else you would like to share that you think will add value to the readers?

I think my best advice is to understand that all of our bodies are different. Diets never work for the long term, the only thing that works is a lifestyle change that suits each of our individual lives. Pay attention, and track how your body responds to certain foods. For some people carbs are the problem, but for me, I can't handle a lot of fats. My body does not handle fats well and they will cause my sugar to spike and remain that way for hours. My diet now consists of fresh fruit and vegetables with very little processed foods. I eat as much as I want, whenever I want, I even have desert every now and then, but I have found that once I got my A1c under control, I am rarely hungry and no longer have the ridiculous cravings that I used to have.

I will occasionally eat a piece of meat, but inevitably will regret it the next day. I am not on a diet, I am not a vegetarian for moral/ethical/religious reasons. I have made a choice to be healthy and this is the lifestyle that I choose because it works best for me. I can choose to be a victim to this disease or I can choose to be victorious in this battle. I refuse to be a victim any longer!

I am a Diabetes Dominator. What about you?

http://www.bobbierobertson.com

SHAWN SHEPHEARD

Question 1: Who are you? What makes you happy? What hobbies are you passionate about? Who do you love? What do you do for a living? Essentially, your bio plus some personal stuff!

My name is Shawn Shepheard. Here's a peek at my crazy ("crazy good," that is) life:

I run a hockey program for children that have never played hockey before called the Slapshot Program, hosted by the Character Community Foundation of York Region.

I love, love, love the generous spirit of the diabetes community and my involvement includes:

Hosting the Sugar Free Shawn Show — we have lots of fun profiling people living well with diabetes, and share tips on how you too can have fun and live well with diabetes.

Keynote Speaking — nothing is better than being in a room full of people that just "get it" regarding diabetes and living life to the fullest. I love presenting to health care providers, and people living with diabetes.

Host of The Sugar Free Shawn Network — I've always wondered how we keep the connection and inspiration going between events, you know day to day, when it's easy to feel like we are all alone. The Network is my answer to keeping that connection and energy alive, every day.

Author — It still feels a little weird calling myself an author, but I am proud to have released my book: 'Life is Sweet'".

Helping Companies that I Love — I've been involved in corporate training for many years.

You know the funny thing? I believe lasting results only happen when leaders work together with their teams, and communicate on an ongoing basis. The answers don't lie with the "expert" who comes in and preaches, then leaves. I call that the supply teacher syndrome, because the team knows you will not be there tomorrow.

In my spare time I love hanging out with my wife, reading, playing hockey (or cheering for my favorite team), and running marathons in support of Team Diabetes.

Question 2: What is your diabetes story? Please share your story of diagnosis and the path you traveled to get where you are today. What have been your biggest struggles/triumphs in regard to living with diabetes? How does diabetes makes you awesome at life? What are the tools you use to manage your diabetes day to day (pump, MDI, CGM, etc.)?

Living with diabetes can really suck --I know, because I live with it every day. But, there is great news: life can be really, really, really sweet.

I was diagnosed with Type One diabetes on Christmas Day 1997. I know first-hand the challenges that those of us living with diabetes face; however, by sharing personal examples and experiences from my own journey, I have inspired many people to push the boundaries of what is possible in their own lives.

I've spoken to thousands of people who are living with diabetes, to those who care for those who have diabetes and everyone in between. I am known for my real, engaging, no BS style, and my dogged determination to make diabetes a lot less scary for people. I share from my experiences and I tell stories that move people to take action to get the life they want to live!

As for the tools I use, I started on the Dexcom G4 Platinum Continuous Glucose Monitor in March 2014. The CGM is a device that provides real-time glucose readings, allowing people with diabetes to see their glucose levels 24/7 and track how quickly our blood sugar levels are increasing or decreasing.

Question 3: What are your top 3 tips for thriving with diabetes that you believe have served you (and continue to serve you) best along your diabetes journey?

My three tips are:

1. Create Your Diabetes Dream Team

    There is a saying that we are the average of the five people we hang out with most often. There is a lot of truth in that. The great news is, we get to choose who we hang out with. Go out and find people that inspire you on and off line. There are tons of great people out there! Not sure where to start? I would suggest looking at local events and get involved, as for online, this book is a great start!

2. Don't Be Too Hard On Yourself

    Diabetes can kick our butts. There will be challenging days, unfortunately that is something we can't avoid. The key, is not to be too hard on ourselves. One of the sayings I repeat to myself when I am having a rough day is: "This too shall pass."

3. Daily Gratitude

    We are surrounded by "bad' news, on newscasts in newspapers and all around us, and it is easy to get caught up in all the negativity. This simple exercise of investing a few minutes each day and writing down what you are truly grateful for in the moment truly shifts our energy and puts us in a good mood.

Question 4: Is there anything else you would like to share that you think will add value to the readers?

Everything starts with a GREAT attitude. It's not so easy to put on that same positive attitude day after day, especially when you're facing challenging times at work or at home regarding health or money.

However, you can choose to be a positive influence to others.

Once you put on your positive attitude in the morning, it's your job to keep it on. Of course you will have bad days and unpleasant things will happen, but it's how you choose to react to these situations that are important. You can acknowledge these events and then let them go, and slip right back into your positive attitude.

The Gem – When you choose to be positive, you will notice and attract more positive things and people into your life.

Your Piggy Bank Payment – Perform a "random act of kindness" to make someone's day.

On the Write Track – Start your own gratitude journal and aim to make an entry every single day. Write about what you're grateful for, and include the things YOU did to make a positive impact on the world.

You can find Shawn's book online:

Life is Sweet: Surviving Diabetes and a Whole Lot of Other Crazy Stuff

www.sugarfreeshawn.com

JODY STANISLAW

Question 1: Who are you? What makes you happy? What hobbies are you passionate about? Who do you love? What do you do for a living? Essentially, your bio plus some personal stuff!

Hello! I'm Jody Stanislaw, Type 1 since 1980, diagnosed when I was 7. What makes me happy? I love that question. It's actually one I pose to my patients often, because if you don't know the answer, life probably isn't very happy. It's a good one to think about. So here I go....I love moving my body via yoga, biking, hiking and more, preferably outside in nature, spending time with friends, laughing, movies, books, healthy and delicious food, taking impeccable care of the planet, sunrises and sunsets, travel and seeing other cultures, being well rested, having a healthy and fit body, taking care of my diabetes and having great numbers, helping others, speaking engagements where I get to inspire the audience, how easily the internet allows me to touch thousands of lives, focusing on gratitude every day, sending birthday cards, soft blankets, naps, roses, breathtaking flower arrangements, sunshine and blue skies, swimming in the ocean, clean water....I could go on and on!

Everything about me is extroverted. I love people. People fascinate me. We are all so different, and everyone has an amazing story. I certainly have a lot of good ones! I love to inspire people. I've reached my dream of becoming a physician, and my next one is to become an inspirational speaker. So, if you'd like to hire me, I'm available!

Being healthy is at the core of who I am, physically as well as mentally. I came from a healthy minded family, both of my parents being very active people to this day, but living with diabetes has certainly played a big role in making me this way as well. I exercise almost daily. It could be my beloved hot yoga class, a hilly bike ride, a steep hike, a day on the ski slopes, cutting up the lake on my waterski, or just a good sweat at the gym. Another yet unfulfilled dream I have is to become a hip hop dancer! Not sure when I'm going to fit that one in though. But, I got 2nd place in a local Dancing With The Stars contest, so perhaps that's a good start!

Question 2: What is your diabetes story? Please share your story of diagnosis and the path you traveled to get where you are today. What have been your biggest struggles/triumphs in regard to living with diabetes? How does diabetes makes you awesome at life? What are the tools you use to manage your diabetes day to day (pump, MDI, CGM, etc.)?

I actually don't remember anything negative about my diagnosis. Sure, I was painfully thirsty for about a week, wet my bed nightly, lost a ton of weight yet was eating like a horse...all the typical symptoms. But after we realized what was going on, I checked into Seattle Children's hospital and had a fun time there for about a week.

Since I wasn't really sick, more just there for education for my family, I ran around the hallways and chatted with everyone I could meet all day long, had my own TV, and made cool stuff in the arts and crafts room. It was a blast. I had so much fun that it was this experience that shaped my decision to want to become a doctor when I grew up.

Once we got home, we cleared out all the sugar in the house and started using measuring cups as serving utensils. Meals were now at exact times, and included exact amounts of food which stayed constant from day to day. I weighed and measured everything I ate. I still have the food and sugar logs I kept from the first few years to this day.

One of the highlights of my childhood with diabetes was going to diabetes summer camp. I was diagnosed in June, and one of the things we learned about at the hospital was this fantastic camp that was coming up in July. I don't know if my parents would have ever even sent me to summer camp had we not learned about this opportunity. So, off I went to diabetes camp in July, and to this day, it's been one of the best experiences of my life.

I went to that camp every summer for 8 years. One of my fellow campers, Missy, became my one and only best friend with diabetes.

She and I would laugh so hard that we'd get in trouble every night. This was of course pre-internet, so she and I would only see each other during that week of the year. The rest of the year we'd write letters. I've tried to find Missy in my adult years, but with a last name like Davis, which by now has probably been replaced by a married name, I've had no luck.

Camp continues to shape my life in positive ways even today. I've been on staff now for several years at diabetes camps in Washington state and Idaho. The ability to give back is priceless, and all the people I've met involved with camps are always amazingly big-hearted, phenomenal people, many of whom have become my closest friends.

As I was growing up, never once do I remember any adult making me feel that diabetes was anything I should feel bad or scared about. My bubbly and positive spirit continued on as I went along with this new way of life. For this, I am immensely grateful. When I see parents today giving a message of pity and fear to their child with diabetes, it breaks my heart. Diabetes is far from a death sentence. It can easily be used as something that gives a level of strength that only living with a chronic disease could ever give. Going through life being taught about nutrition, the importance of exercise, gaining discipline, responsibility, and tenacity, along with the message that we can do anything we want and live a long, healthy, happy life is available to everyone with diabetes.

Now, having said that, I certainly don't mean to imply that living with diabetes hasn't also been extremely challenging and scary at times. I don't remember exactly when my excitement for this new thing that I got a lot of attention for turned, but what I do remember is starting to secretly binge on sugar.

I knew where the cookie jar was at all of my friends' houses. Anytime I'd do a sleep over and everyone was asleep, I'd tip-toe into their kitchen so I could eat some cookies. Grandma always had sugary granola on the top shelf of the pantry, and when I got lucky, she'd also have ice cream in the freezer. Anytime I was at her house, I'd wait until everyone seemed busy and sneak into the kitchen to indulge. My heart would race for fear I'd get caught.

This habit turned into a binging disorder in my teens that lasted for years. It got so bad in my twenties that it was truly consuming my life. I broke down in tears one day at my best friend Jen's house, and she helped me find an inpatient eating disorder rehab center. I flew down to Arizona shortly after, and stayed there for two months.

I'd love to say that all of that is behind me now, but that is not the truth. Having to watch every single bite of food that enters my mouth and wonder what it's going to do to my blood sugar levels day after day for me is very taxing. I dream about a cure, not so I don't have to do shots or poke my finger anymore, but to be relieved of this daily burden. Gratefully however, I truly enjoy eating an extremely healthy diet now, and making healthy decisions I'd say about 90% of the time. The basis of my diet is low carb, with the bulk of my meals being protein and vegetables, which has given me an A1c between 5.5% and 6% for the past decade.

When I give those numbers, people often ask me about lows. I've only had 3 lows needing assistance in my entire life. I am grateful that I can feel them and also that, as of last year, I got a life-changing CGM. I wore a pump for 5 years, and was even a sales rep for Disetronic pumps for a few years, but I prefer shots. My numbers stay great and I prefer not to be attached to anything. The CGM port doesn't bother me because I put it on my low back and barely remember it's there.

At the age of 42, I'm one of the healthiest women I know. I thank diabetes for this. I thank diabetes for motivating me to make healthy food choices. I thank diabetes for inspiring me to make exercise an integral part of my life. I thank diabetes for the strength and tenacity I have built from all the times I've struggled and wanted to give up, but didn't. I thank diabetes for my ability to relate to and touch others who are struggling with intense physical and emotional issues. I thank diabetes for teaching me that I can conquer anything. I thank diabetes for driving me to always make lemonade when life hands me lemons. And finally, I thank diabetes for generating my passion to make a career out of helping others live healthier lives.

My childhood dream came true at the age of 35, when I graduated from medical school and was finally announced as Dr. Jody Stanislaw. Today, I work with many types of patients, but of course specialize in Type 1. Being able to pass my life-changing wisdom on for how to manage this disease to others via phone or Skype, wisdom which took me decades of frustrating trials and tribulations to figure out on my own, is one of the greatest joys of my life.

After 35 years of living with what could be a devastating disease, yet being as healthy as I am, is a great tool in itself to bring hope to anyone living with T1D, especially to families with a child with Type 1, and to any patient feeling doomed by this disease. I have the personal experience plus formal education to help patients out of their struggles, and to instill them with life-saving education, plus hope and inspiration. So if you are reading this and would like to have a chat, give me a call! I'd love to help, and I'd love to remind you how awesome you are. **www.ConsultWithDrJody.com/Type1** or **www.DrJodyND.com**

Question 3: What are your top 3 tips for thriving with diabetes that you believe have served you (and continue to serve you) best along your diabetes journey?

Take Care of Your Body
When you feel good, you can conquer the world. When you don't, endless opportunities pass you by. You have one exciting life to live, and the one precious vehicle to carry you through this exciting ride called Your Life is your body.

See the Cup Half Full
Curve balls happen. The plans you have will fall apart. Rain will pour on your picnic. Your friend will forget to call you back. Your spouse will irritate you. But guess what? You're not alone. These things happens to everyone. These events are part of life. Let this stuff go, and focus on the good.

Know What Makes You Happy and Make Time for It

This is your life. What kind of person do you want to be? What fills your heart with joy and satisfaction? Are you doing that? Make time for what makes you happy and boldly go for it.

Live by the 80/20 Rule

Perfection is a low expectation because it's impossible. It sucks up energy. Perfection = pure fiction. The rule I teach all of my patients to live by, and that I follow as well, is the 80/20 rule. Make healthy eating choices 80% of the time. Indulge 20% of the time and enjoy it. Let go of perfection.

You can find Jody's book online:

Hunger: An Adventurous Journey of Finding Peace Within

www.DrJodyND.com

www.ConsultWithDrJody.com/Type1

MIKE SUANN

Question 1: Who are you? What makes you happy? What hobbies are you passionate about? Who do you love? What do you do for a living? Essentially, your bio plus some personal stuff!

My name is Mike Suann. Things that make me happy are my family, my wife and children. I have some very close mates, and we enjoy motorcycle riding together. We love exploring our country on two wheels, and experiencing everything our country has to offer. Like most people I enjoy my music, watching movies and TV, getting out for a bite to eat or a walk along the beach. I work for Qantas as a Licensed Aircraft Maintenance Engineer. I have moved up through the ranks to now be in Maintenance Operations Control. We oversee our aircraft on the ground undergoing maintenance and in flight, and directly talk with the flight crew when they are operating the aircraft on many and various flights. My work involves 24/7 shiftwork, and I work 12 hour shifts. This poses many issues for a T1D, but I manage it as I enjoy the lifestyle my shiftwork provides.

Question 2: What is your diabetes story? Please share your story of diagnosis and the path you traveled to get where you are today. What have been your biggest struggles/triumphs in regard to living with diabetes? How does diabetes makes you awesome at life? What are the tools you use to manage your diabetes day to day (pump, MDI, CGM, etc.)?

I am 48 years old and have lived with type 1 diabetes (T1D) for 30 years this October. My "dia-versary" is October 25th, 1985. During my Year 11 studies at school, I had to do an assignment on a disease and chose diabetes as my father had type 2 diabetes, so I was familiar with the symptoms. Little did I know that 2 years later, I was to be diagnosed with type 1. Six months into the 1st year of my apprenticeship, I felt the symptoms of unquenchable thirst, constant fatigue, and extreme weight loss. I knew something was wrong, and went to my GP hoping above all hope that he would say I had a virus or flu or something that wasn't a chronic disease such as diabetes. I was in shock when he tested my blood sugar and it was 33 mmol. He told me to go home and get my parents to take me straight to the emergency ward at Sutherland Hospital.

The rest is history, with needles twice a day, long acting and short acting insulin, mixing both in a syringe, watching what I was eating (most of the time), etc. I am now on a pump, and sometimes use Continuous Glucose Monitor. However, at a cost of $70 per sensor that only lasts for 6 days with no rebate or refund from my health fund or the NDSS (National Diabetes Supplies Scheme), it is financially impossible to use a sensor every day of the year for me. I rarely have low blood sugars, and those that I do I can treat myself. Life hasn't always been this easy, as once upon a time I was on needles up to 3 times a day using short and/or long acting to control my blood sugars. When I was first diagnosed, I was on porcine insulin (derived from pigs), and when I was on this insulin I could easily feel a low coming on... the cold sweats, the shakes. But, mentally I was still with it and thus relied on no-one but myself to get me out of the low with juice. Then, I was told the production of porcine insulin in Australia would be withdrawn, and was to be replaced with artificial human insulin. This was supposed to be the "bees' knees" of new treatment for T1D. Not long after (by that I mean within days), I no longer had any indications of a low coming on, so before I knew it, I was a blithering idiot with people wondering if I was drunk at work or just sleepy because I came to work with little sleep from partying all night. Wrong!!! My blood sugar was low! No one can understand how scary and extremely embarrassing this experience is unless they have been through it themselves.

I also believe that the mood swings associated with having high or low blood sugars also contributed to the failure of my first marriage. This, along with shiftwork, depression due to this chronic disease, loss of loved ones, and the other stressors of life ultimately culminated in my divorce from the mother of my children. I have moved on, and am in a great place now with my new wife who has an excellent understanding of and empathy for my T1D. We are true soul mates, and enjoy life greatly together. I was diagnosed with heart disease on April Fool's Day 2014 at the age of 46. What a shock! When riding my push bike for some exercise, I started feeling some chest pain. I didn't really pay much attention to it, however, after getting the same pain at the same point in my ride for the 3rd time in a row, I figured something wasn't right. After another fateful trip to my GP and a Cardiologist, it was discovered that one of my arteries was 80% blocked and I needed a stent inserted to relieve the condition. Along with this artery, there were others that were significantly affected, so a treatment of aspirin and other heart medication was commenced, and now I take aspirin daily to keep my blood thin and to prevent further complications. During my previous 28 years living with diabetes, my cholesterol had always been in a good range, so this alone is not the only predictor of heart disease. Both of my parents suffered from heart disease in their later years as well, so this is more likely the origin of my heart disease.

Question 3: What are your top 3 tips for thriving with diabetes that you believe have served you (and continue to serve you) best along your diabetes journey?

• Don't let diabetes define you. Do what you want, what makes you happy. Of course, you have to make some exceptions and adjustments, but make these all part of it and enjoy your journey.

• Maintain a balance. Don't rule out eating sweets or make a list of things that "you can't eat." As long as you maintain a balance, life is good!

• Always be conscious of where you are mentally. By that I mean take five, and ask yourself some questions: How am I doing today? Am I in a good place? What is upsetting me? Why am I getting frustrated? What is making me feel great? Why am I angry? Some days you'll have different answers to all these questions, and that is okay and to be expected. Deal with it and move on, but always be conscious of where you are in the current moment.

Question 4: Is there anything else you would like to share that you think will add value to the readers?

I am continually amazed how well I can function when my blood sugar is going low. Normal blood sugar levels are anywhere between 4.5 to 6.5 mmol for a person without diabetes. Sometimes, I can test my blood sugar and be as low as 2.8 mmol, and still feel like I am functioning normally. Only someone who knows me really well could tell. In 1985 when I was first diagnosed, my glucometer was the size of a house brick. It ran on 4 'AA' batteries, and every time I used it I had to calibrate it. The time it took to test was 2 minutes, 1 minute to leave a drop of blood on the test strip, then wipe it off and leave it for another minute to develop and then test it under the light source in the glucometer. Now, I can test my blood sugar on my iPhone with my Dario glucometer which is the size of an eraser. When using my CGM, I can know exactly what my blood sugars are doing every 5 minutes. This development for diabetes management is truly liberating. Shame it isn't cheap enough to use continually, then life would really be a breeze.

One more thing that comes to mind is that depending on what mood I'm in when I go low, that affects what type of low blood sugar experience I have. By that I mean if I am happy and I end up low, I am super happy and it is like I'm on a happiness drug. When I am grumpy or down and end up low, I can be extremely angry or even furious. Again, this is an example of the mood swings that diabetes can cause related to our blood sugar levels. Lastly, my T1D has had a huge impact on my life, and I feel as though I wouldn't be the same person if I never had diabetes. Although I have type 1 diabetes, this does not define me!

GINGER VIEIRA

Question 1: Who are you? What makes you happy? What hobbies are you passionate about? Who do you love? What do you do for a living? Essentially, your bio plus some personal stuff!

My name is Ginger Vieira and I'm a lady who loves to write, loves dogs, loves movies, and loves small gatherings with one or three of my favorite people versus huge groups. I've known I wanted to be a writer (or that I *am* a writer) since the 2nd grade. While I've taken an awesome unexpected detour into the health and fitness realm—I set 15 records in drug-free powerlifting between 2009 and 2011, with record lifts of 308 lb. deadlift, 265 lb. squat, and 190 lb. bench press in the women's 148 lb. weight-class—I'm still really a writer at heart. I'm grateful to be able to *write* about health and fitness today as the Editor at DiabetesDaily.com, but I also *love* to write books. To some it sounds like a torturous, horrible idea, but to me, the process of filling those pages feels exactly like what my brain was designed to do. So far I have written "Your Diabetes Science Experiment," "Emotional Eating with Diabetes," and "Dealing with Diabetes Burnout."

Today, I live in the woods of Vermont with my handsome husband, my gorgeous baby daughter, and our ridiculous canine pack, Blue, Petey, and Einstein.

Update: during the publishing process of this book, Einstein has sadly crossed over the rainbow bridge and is now in the canine clouds. He will be sorely missed and forever in our hearts.

Question 2: What is your diabetes story? Please share your story of diagnosis and the path you traveled to get where you are today. What have been your biggest struggles/triumphs in regard to living with diabetes? How does diabetes makes you

awesome at life? What are the tools you use to manage your diabetes day to day (pump, MDI, CGM, etc.)?

Oh, diabetes stories are so much fun! Ahh, just kidding. I was 13 years old and everyone in my family got the flu…but my flu never went away. In fact, it just got worse, and weirder. All the classic symptoms developed within 3 weeks: extreme thirst (standing at the bathroom sink at 3 a.m. scooping water into my mouth), lots of peeing, weight-loss (but I was 13, maybe weight-loss was just puberty…right?), blurry vision (but everyone in my family had glasses…so probably just my time…right?), and extreme fatigue in my legs (but telling my mom I didn't want to go to school isn't that alarming from a 13 year old!).

A week later, I saw this poster in my science class with all the symptoms of diabetes and I knew that's what I had. I told my mom and she said, "No, that's impossible! Old people get that!" A few days later I started crying because I felt so lousy. We went to the doctor and the rest is history!

A big part of my "diabetes story" is going from a junior in college who had sat on her butt for a year as the Editor of the college newspaper, feeling very unhealthy, eating junk, very little exercise….to a senior in college who was getting certified in Ashtanga yoga (power yoga), training in powerlifting, and getting certified as a personal trainer (while finishing college with a degree in Professional Writing).

What I learned during the next few years while competing in powerlifting, setting records I never planned on setting, and really *feeling* like an athlete will always impact how I take care of my diabetes for the rest of my life. In the tiniest nutshell possible: I learned that there's a physiological reason behind every blood sugar. I learned how to *fuel* my body with real food. I learned just how powerful my body is, whether or not I'm powerlifting. I learned how to connect to my body with pride instead of feeling like the girl with several chronic illnesses. I learned how to feel powerful, both physically and mentally. Period. And while I don't train in powerlifting now and certainly don't have any of that intense strength, I still feel powerful.

Question 3: What are your top 3 tips for thriving with diabetes that you believe have served you (and continue to serve you) best along your diabetes journey?

1. Don't make excuses: ask for answers…and go find them! One of the easiest ways to spend the rest of your life frustrated by your blood sugars is to believe that they are random and irrational. Every blood sugar has a cause and a reason—some of those causes we can't control, but we can plan differently for them. Your body's physiology is not random! Seek answers…it's worth it!

2. Diabetes sucks—there's no arguing with that—and I think letting yourself express your diabetes frustrations is really important, and really healthy. You can take excellent care of your diabetes and still shout from the rooftops that it sucks to deal with every day. Express it! Don't let those emotions get all clogged up in your heart and soul and mind, preventing you from being able to take care of yourself.

3. The moment we acknowledge how much *what we eat* impacts our blood sugars and our ability to manage our blood sugars, the easier diabetes management will become. But that doesn't mean you have to eat perfectly or go the rest of your life without dessert. Just make room for that dessert by focusing most of your nutrition on eating whole, clean foods (mostly veggies, good quality protein and fats, etc.)…and then have some damn dessert! You don't have to be perfect in order to succeed.

Question 4: Is there anything else you would like to share that you think will add value to the readers?

Figure out what scares you…and go do it! I'm not talking about getting locked into a closet full of spiders…but the things you'd love to achieve but are afraid of pursuing. Do them. The more you're afraid of succeeding in that dream, the more rewarding it will be when you go after it. (And of course, if at first you don't succeed, just keep trying, damnit!)

You can find Ginger's books online:

Your Diabetes Science Experiment

Emotional Eating with Diabetes

Dealing with Diabetes Burnout

www.diabetesdaily.com

LIS WARREN

Question 1: Who are you? What makes you happy? What hobbies are you passionate about? Who do you love? What do you do for a living? Essentially, your bio plus some personal stuff!

My name is Lis Warren. I was born in England, but am half Danish. I trained as a pianist and music teacher in London. I've recently retired from the UK's Civil Service, where over the years I worked on music education, school health, special educational needs, and school food policy. I now volunteer on many different diabetes-related projects including local clinical commissioning, the National Health Service Diabetes Patient Experience group, Diabetes UK, and I take part in as many diabetes research programs that will take me! I love to walk in the countryside, to sing, to go to jazz, classical, opera and salsa concerts, to dance salsa, take photos, and to travel. Sunny days and a glass of wine with friends or family make me happy – as does witnessing the appreciation shown by any person with diabetes who gets help via the Diabetes Online Community (#DOC)!

Question 2: What is your diabetes story? Please share your story of diagnosis and the path you traveled to get where you are today. What have been your biggest struggles/triumphs in regard to living with diabetes? How does diabetes makes you awesome at life? What are the tools you use to manage your diabetes day to day (pump, MDI, CGM, etc.)?

I was diagnosed at age 13 in 1965, after a short period of experiencing what we call the 4 T's in the UK: thirst, toilet, tiredness, thin. I spent 2-3 weeks in hospital learning how to measure carbs - I was told to eat 200g each day at set times (in 6 portions – so lots of snacks) and to take fixed insulin doses. Blood sugar levels took around 3 hours to be tested (and could not be done at home), and the HbA1c test did not exist. I tested my urine with a tablet in a test tube that would fizz and spit until it turned blue (negative), greenish, or orange (4+ meaning a high blood sugar). I've no real idea how my control was, but I don't recall frequent hypos at school so I guess my blood sugars were pretty high for most of the time. Diabetes education did not exist, and I saw my doctor once or twice a year for the first few decades post-diagnosis. I just got on with it, and diabetes never figured very high on my list of priorities, though it's now clear to me how it's affected my character in the long run.

I developed some retinopathy in my late 20s which was successfully treated with laser therapy, and has thankfully remained totally stable since then. I've never knowingly had DKA, though I've twice been in hospital due firstly to a stubborn infection, then what I suspect was considered poor control in my teenage years, but these weren't emergencies. Other than regular hospital appointments, I've only missed a single day's work due directly to diabetes when I had a very severe night hypo (when my husband was abroad) and didn't come round until 4pm!

My biggest diabetes-related struggle relates to eating behaviors. I recall being told at 13 that I could never eat sweets (candies) again, plus the slavish weighing and measuring of food very quickly got to me in the early days. I became obsessed with what I ate, and began a lifelong struggle with my weight - what we call yo-yo dieting - which clearly affected my diabetes management, causing both highs and lows, and a poor HbA1c. I think it went up to around 9.4 in my late 20s. My weight fluctuated a lot, and I often discussed my feelings about this with doctors, but as I was never severely under or over weight in their eyes, it was over 40 years with type 1 and chaotic eating before I got to see an eating disorders specialist. I then finally made my peace with food, stopped using it to help manage my emotions, and reached a place of total freedom about how and what I eat.

As a youngster, I was never really afraid of having type 1, possibly because it was never (seemingly at least!) made into a big issue by anyone I had contact with. Nobody told me I'd die early or warned me not to do stuff. I was a keen horse rider; I love snorkeling and diving, and have always done everything I wanted to do in life. On reflection, I think having type 1 has given me incredible resilience, an ability to cope with challenges, and the self-reliance that's needed to get the most from life. Some might say I'm verging on foolhardy, and I do of course have wonderful support from my husband, who has rescued me from many severe hypos (pre CGM – THE best innovation in my 50 years with type 1), and reminds me constantly to carry emergency supplies! But, the hard work I've put in over many decades of growing up with diabetes has, I believe, given me a very positive and accepting attitude towards living with it, so much so that I now embrace diabetes and its physical *and* emotional characteristics. It deserves my love, care and attention.

I started using CGM in 2013, which was like switching a light on in a dark cave, and after 48 years of injections, I finally started pumping insulin in 2014. I use an integrated pump with CGM (Animas Vibe*) and this combo has transformed and hugely improved my diabetes management skills. I now have the best HbA1c I've ever had, and I'm really proud of this in my 50th year of having type 1! I've received two 50 year medals, one from Diabetes UK and one from Joslin, and I spend most of my time campaigning for better services and supporting those who need information to live well with their diabetes. I'm certainly no saint, and I make many mistakes and occasional misjudgments, but it's a hugely rewarding activity as I continue to learn things every single day, whilst hopefully helping others who are at the start of their diabetes journey.

Question 3: What are your top 3 tips for thriving with diabetes that you believe have served you (and continue to serve you) best along your diabetes journey?

- Volunteer for research. Taking part helps you learn lots of new stuff about diabetes, provides a massive boost to your motivation to manage things well, and you also meet the most wonderful clinicians and researchers who are doing really interesting things to help us all. Some studies involve medical examinations, so you may get a 'check over' that's not normally available via standard channels. If any group work or discussion is involved, you may also get the chance to meet lots of other people with diabetes, which is great fun! And of course, you'll be helping others farther down the line, so everybody wins.

- Feel your anger and sadness at diagnosis, talk it through and express your feelings, seek professional psychological support if needed, *but then move on*. Don't blame diabetes for everything that's tough in your life – you'll give it a bad name! Make it your friend, your baby within that you care for, love and cherish as you do any other physical feature you own. It saddens me greatly to read of diabetes as the 'devil' – you can't live happily with a devil on your back, so this depiction can't be helpful. You can't fight diabetes, as it will always win. To achieve peace and happiness, you must make it your friend and look after it, then dump your anger and put your energy into enjoying the fun things in life!

- Join the Diabetes Online Community (#DOC). There is more than enough education and information out there! There are Facebook groups on every diabetes topic under the sun, diabetes Tweet Chats every week in many different countries and in many languages – and if it doesn't exist, you can create it! Any need for quick info or support can be satisfied 24/7 without waiting for a clinic appointment in 6 months' time, but do use your judgment. Avoid sites that are negative, stay with the winners, and if you're uncertain, check out medical advice with your own doctor or nurse. I've made friends online all over the world, and have now met many of them in person at diabetes events. It's a wonderful community, and is full of great role models who will inspire and support, especially if you're struggling. It really is the best club to join, and most people with diabetes have a fantastic sense of humor!

Twitter: @liswarren

Guest Blog Post:

https://grumpypumper.wordpress.com/2014/04/30/loving-and-learning-from-the-doc-diabetes-online-community/

RACHEL ZINMAN

Question 1: Who are you? What makes you happy? What hobbies are you passionate about? Who do you love? What do you do for a living? Essentially, your bio plus some personal stuff!

My name is Rachel Zinman, and I'm 49 years old. I live in Australia, but I wasn't born here. I was born in Holland to American parents. I'm officially American, but I only "officially" lived there for 11 years. I've spent over 30 years in Australia. I discovered Yoga when I was 19, and I love it. It's what makes me sing. It's my passion, my work, and my hobby all in one. I've had lots of other incarnations as a dancer, mother, Waldorf educator, award winning musician, published writer, and poet. But for me, Yoga is it. If it weren't for Yoga I'm sure all those other things wouldn't have had the same meaning. In fact, Yoga has enabled me to see the meaningfulness in and through every pursuit in my life.

Question 2: What is your diabetes story? Please share your story of diagnosis and the path you traveled to get where you are today. What have been your biggest struggles/triumphs in regard to living with diabetes? How does diabetes makes you awesome at life? What are the tools you use to manage your diabetes day to day (pump, MDI, CGM, etc.)?

My story of diagnosis and acceptance has been a long one. Up until the age of 42, all my blood tests had been normal, but I was having unusual symptoms as early as 2001. Both doctors and alternative health practitioners mentioned I had the symptoms of diabetes, but because it didn't show up on my blood tests, there was no cause for concern. Then at 42, everything changed. I collapsed, couldn't get out of bed, and eating sugar made me feel panicky and dizzy. My husband forced me to have a blood test, my fasting sugar was slightly

high, and my A1c was over 6. My doctor shoved a whole bunch of
pamphlets at me, and told me to google diabetes. He said I'd have to
work out how to cure it. The guy was a moron and I never went
back! Luckily, I found an amazing endocrinologist. At first we
thought it was type 2, or maybe just an endocrine imbalance. He
suggested I manage it with diet and lifestyle. I wasn't overweight, and
was super healthy and disciplined, so he was sure we could reverse
things. So, for a while, I managed it well. I never bothered to read
about my condition. Just ate, exercised, and checked my blood sugar
once or twice a day. A year later, things were good, but he wanted to
do an antibody test just in case. The results weren't good. He told me
my body was attacking itself. He never mentioned I might have type
1, but he did say medication was inevitable. I refused to believe him.
For 6 years I worked hard to keep my levels low. I ate less and less
carbs, marched up and down hills, but I just felt more and more
depleted. I went to acupuncturists, ayurvedic therapists,
kineseologists, I did tapping, yoga chanting, made flower mandalas,
you name it I tried it. But things kept getting worse. I kept thinking,
soon it will change, soon I'll get better. Yogis don't get diabetes! But
eventually, I developed neuropathy, my digestion was terrible, and I'd
lost a ton of weight. My morning fasting levels were between 15 and
20 mmol. It was time to haul my butt back to the endo! I'll never
forget the look on his face when he told me I had LADA type 1
diabetes, and it was time to start insulin. I was so scared! I had to wait
a week to start injecting, and I must have cried a river. I think that's
when I really accepted what was happening. There was no going
back. I swear I nearly fainted when I took my first injection in the
CDE's office. My partner was there with me. He told me to breathe.
I started with basal insulin. So far it's been a year. I inject once a day,
and I've been able to reduce my dose to a very small amount. I am
feeling so much better. I've put on weight, have my energy back, and
my whole attitude towards allopathic medicine has shifted. Before my
diagnosis, I was afraid to take a Tylenol. Now, I see how important
proper diagnosis and medication is. I don't regret the choices I made,

but if I'd known sooner that insulin helps preserve beta cells and that it's an absolute lifesaver, I would have started sooner. I totally believed all the myths that are out there about diabetes, and never looked at the hard facts. It's been a real eye opener, and something I don't hesitate to share with anyone I come across who's just been diagnosed. My daily life and its routines hasn't changed much. I practice Yoga every day twice a day, and eat simple, low carb meals with plenty of leafy green veggies. I eat to live rather than live to eat.

Question 3: What are your top 3 tips for thriving with diabetes that you believe have served you (and continue to serve you) best along your diabetes journey?

- 1. Be kind to myself, and see the beauty in each moment-don't measure my health by the numbers on my glucometer. Every day is perfect just as it is.

- 2. Yoga, Yoga and more Yoga. Yoga helps me breathe better, feel better, and have the best attitude no matter what the day presents

- 3. Accept what has been given to me, and be grateful. Every single thing I have to share has come from the acceptance of my diagnosis. Accepting that I can never understand why this body has a disease, and knowing that I can never be the disease. But, having it empowers me to make healthy choices. I am sure I'll live a long time because of it.

- **Question 4: Is there anything else you would like to share that you think will add value to the readers?**

When I was first diagnosed I went to visit a friend whose son had been type 1 since he was 8. He taught me how to use my glucometer, and I watched him inject. He was so relaxed about the whole thing. And, there was never a feeling that he was any different to anyone else. Having friends who also live with diabetes is a major plus. That's why I love the diabetes online community, and all the support groups. It's a great way to come to terms with it all. It's a gift!

www.instagram.com/yogafordiabetesblog

www.yogafordiabetesblog.com

www.facebook.com/yogafordiabetesblog

www.rachelzinmanyoga.com

https://www.youtube.com/user/Rachelakshmi

Daniele Hargenrader

PART SIX - DIABETES DOMINATOR RESOURCES

A DIABETES DOMINATOR NEVER STOPS LEARNING

BLOGS

"The time is always right to do the right thing."
-Martin Luther King, Jr.

Don't let your low blood sugars make your weight and A1c high!

When you're a nine-year-old kid, the word "diabetes" is not generally a familiar one
—or at least it wasn't to me. To me, it meant a world of change in the blink of an eye. It meant going from being a "regular kid" to one with a chronic disease that would require constant, around-the-clock monitoring of food intake, injections, and blood sugar checks. It meant not being a "regular" kid anymore. These feelings are true of anyone who is diagnosed with diabetes, no matter what age it happens.

One of the things that tend to happen as a person with diabetes develops their protocols on daily management is a specific thing we eat or drink when our blood sugar gets low. Now, for some people, this has always been juice and there is nothing else to it. However, for me and for many of the people with diabetes I've worked with, having a low blood sugar was an excuse to have some kind of treat. And not just a little bit of a treat; it was usually a huge portion of that treat, plus some other things as well. For me, it ranged anywhere from Skittles to a big bowl of Cocoa Pebbles with milk (if I only knew then what I know now!), to a big bagel with melted cheese, and anything else unhealthy you could think of. And it would not be the serving size required to treat my low blood sugar! It was always at least double or triple the amount that would have been needed, and that, my friends, packed on the pounds!

So after many years of "treating" myself when my blood sugar was low, I finally realized what a detriment to my health it had become. I also noticed how often my blood sugar levels were fluctuating from low to very high afterward, the blood sugar rollercoaster. With the giant portions of carbs I was eating to treat the low blood sugar, I was always over-treating, which would lead to high blood sugar an hour later. This then required more insulin, and more insulin allows more fat storage on the body, and you can see the vicious cycle that I had going on. With a hemoglobin A1c of 13.5% at its highest, and being considered obese on the height/weight measurement scale at 200 pounds, eventually I realized I was going about taking care of my diabetes the wrong way.

The human brain is an amazing thing, and when we train it to know that a treat is coming when our blood sugar is low, we are subconsciously training ourselves to have more low blood sugars than we would if we were just using 100% juice boxes, glucose gel, or glucose tabs and never anything else. Low blood sugar is horrible for our brains and every other part of our internal environment. Go stock up on 100% juice boxes, glucose tabs, and glucose gel. Learn from my mistakes, friends: don't "treat" low blood sugars with junk food. Bad habits are tough to break!

Finding inspiration and fulfillment by choosing to make diabetes a strength instead of a weakness.

Now that I have had T1D for 24 years and have had the experience of living with it through childhood, adolescence, teens, 20s, and now 30s, I can say with certainty that it is finally okay with ME that I have diabetes. If you would've asked me about my experience with diabetes ten or 15 years ago, my response would not have been a positive one, as it is now. I might have told you about how much work it is, or how hard it is to live with it, or how much I hated it, or a variety of other mainly self-pity-driven descriptions of how I felt, and they all would have been the truth at that time. Truth be told, feeling that way all the time sucked—like really sucked—and I'm sure I'm not the only one who experienced or is still experiencing these feelings towards their diabetes.

If you ask me now about my experience with diabetes, I would tell you that it is the card I have been dealt, and I have learned to play it to my advantage, much like any other perceived disadvantage can become an advantage if we change our perceptions, or the meanings we give things and experiences. Before, it was like I was alone in this diabetes world and nobody understood what it was like to be me. I had T1D for 15 years before I even met anyone else who had diabetes; and even then, I barely knew that person and unfortunately didn't put forth the effort to get to know them better. I continued on through my 20s, occasionally meeting others with diabetes; but again, I never really sat down and had a conversation with anyone specifically about what it was like living with diabetes from their perspective.

Fast-forward to the present, where it is my passion, my career, and my true mission in life to help other people with diabetes by teaching them the systems I have developed over the years that have allowed me to consistently have a hemoglobin A1c level below 6.5%, and has also allowed me to be in the best physical shape of my life. The experiences I get to have with my clients add intense fulfillment to my life; I honestly learn as much from them as they do from me. Ten years ago, I would not have had a very clear picture of my future, and whatever picture I did have wasn't filled with positivity and optimal health. Now when I look into my future, I see only possibilities, opportunities, and experiences that will make me a better, more understanding and accepting person who is always learning, growing, contributing, and adding value to life for myself and others. Changing our perspective is a choice that we all have the ability to make. Anything is possible. Change is good. Change is the price of survival.

Have you made peace with your diabetes? Are you still looking for the way to make it okay? Leave a comment below and let me know where you are in regards to your relationship with your diabetes.

Find more blog posts at diabetesdominator.com

RECIPES

"I am who I am today because of the choices I made yesterday."
-Eleanor Roosevelt

In this section, I've included some of my favorite go-to, super simple, and easy-to-prepare recipes that are all full of nutrient-dense ingredients. If there is an ingredient or seasoning that you don't like, never be afraid to modify! These are just guidelines that are yours to make your own.

That's one thing about cooking that I love so much—as long as you like the way it tastes, then you did it right, whether you followed the directions exactly or not. When it comes to baking, following the directions exactly becomes more important, since baking is more of an exact science; but regular cooking is an art that is open for the artistic interpretation of the artist who is creating the final product!

Diabetes Domintor Basic Smoothie Recipe:

- Big handful of baby spinach/kale/leafy green of choice
- 1/2 cup – 1 cup berries/fruit of choice
- 1 scoop favorite protein powder
- 12 ounces of water or unsweetened nut/seed milk of choice (coconut, almond, flax, hemp), or half water half nut/seed milk
- 1/4 cup full fat Native Forest Unsweetened Coconut Milk (can) OR 1-2 tablespoons peanut or almond butter OR 1/2 avocado
- 1/4 teaspoon stevia if you like it sweeter
- 2 large ice cubes

Optional Add-Ins:

- 1 teaspoon - 1 tablespoon chia/flax/hemp seeds
- 1/2 teaspoon cinnamon
- 1 tablespoon unsweetened cocoa powder

- 1 teaspoon/1 serving fiber supplement

Directions:

I use a Nutribullet blender and put all ingredients into the biggest cup and blend. This recipe will work in any high-speed blender. Just put all ingredients in, blend until all ingredients are fully incorporated, and enjoy!

Overnight No-Cook Chia Seed Breakfast Porridge:

- 2/3 cup chia seeds
- 2 cups unsweetened nut/seed milk of choice (I like to use the vanilla flavored version when available unsweetened coconut/almond/flax/hemp)
- 1/2 teaspoon pure vanilla extract (Frontier brand is alcohol free)
- Stevia to taste

Optional Add-Ins:

- Top with fruit/nuts/unsweetened shredded coconut when ready to serve

Directions:

1. Put chia seeds, nut/seed milk of choice, and vanilla extract in a 1-quart glass jar with a lid.
2. Tighten the lid and shake well to thoroughly combine. Or, stir together seeds, non-dairy milk of choice and vanilla extract in a bowl.
3. Refrigerate overnight.
4. When ready to serve, stir well. Spoon into bowls and top with fruit, nuts and/or coconut if desired. Enjoy!

Spinach Bacon Onion Frittata:

- 1 tablespoon coconut oil or extra-virgin olive oil
- 1 small yellow onion, thinly sliced (about 1 cup)
- 2 cups frozen spinach (from two 10-ounce packages), thawed and squeezed dry
- Celtic sea salt or Real Salt and ground pepper to taste
- 8 large organic/pastured eggs, lightly beaten
- 1/2 cup cooked uncured bacon, crumbled (about 5 slices)

Directions:

1. Preheat oven to 425 degrees Fahrenheit.
2. In a 10-inch ovenproof nonstick skillet, heat oil over medium-high. Add onion and spinach, season with salt and pepper, and cook until onion is translucent, about 5 minutes.
3. Add eggs and bacon, season with salt and pepper, and stir to combine.
4. Cook, undisturbed, until edges are set, about 2 minutes.
5. Transfer skillet to oven and bake until top of frittata is just set, 10 to 13 minutes.
6. Invert or slide frittata onto a plate and cut into 6 wedges. Serve warm or at room temperature!

Slow Cooker Philly Chili:

- 1/4 cup almond or extra virgin olive oil
- 2 medium/large onions, diced
- 2 green bell peppers, seeded and chopped
- 2 red bell peppers, seeded and chopped
- 1 jalapeno, diced
- 3 cloves garlic, minced
- 2 cans black beans, drained and rinsed (please choose low sodium)
- 1 - 26 ounce package Pomi chopped tomatoes OR 2 (15 ounce) cans crushed or diced tomatoes (please choose low sodium if using cans)
- 1 - 6 ounce can tomato paste (low sodium)

- 1 pound organic/grass fed meat of choice, or extra firm organic tofu, or choose to leave it out completely
- Celtic sea salt or Real salt and ground black pepper to taste
- 2 tablespoons ground coriander
- 2 tablespoons Mrs. Dash Fiesta Lime seasoning
- 2 tablespoons dried oregano or Italian seasoning
- 1 tablespoons onion powder
- 1 tablespoon garlic powder

Directions:

1. Heat the oil in a large skillet or soup pot over medium-high heat. Add the onions and all peppers; stir until they start to become soft, about 5 minutes.
2. Add the garlic and season with salt and pepper. Cook and stir until all vegetables are lightly browned, about 10 minutes.
3. If you are using meat, brown grass fed ground beef or diced organic chicken in a separate skillet for about 10 minutes.
4. Add all ingredients into the slow cooker, then add the black beans, tomatoes, tomato paste, and all seasonings into the slow cooker, stir well to combine, and set to the "LOW" setting. Cook on "LOW" for 6-8 hours depending on strength of slow cooker. Enjoy!

White Bean Mashed Potatoes:

- 2 cans low sodium white beans, drained and rinsed thoroughly
- 1 medium shallot, diced
- 2 cloves of garlic, diced
- 1/2 cup – 1 cup of low sodium vegetable or chicken stock or broth (depending on thickness desired, more stock for thinner, less for thicker)
- 1-2 tablespoons Kerrygold grass fed butter or ghee (to taste)
- 1 tablespoon almond oil or extra virgin olive oil
- Celtic Sea Salt or Real salt, pepper, garlic powder, and onion powder to taste

Heat a sauté pan on the stove over medium heat and add almond or extra virgin olive oil, shallots, and garlic. Sauté stirring frequently for about 5 minutes. Add the drained and rinsed beans, vegetable/chicken stock, a pinch of salt, and black or white pepper, garlic powder, and onion powder to the pan, allowing it to simmer gently together for another 5 minutes. Turn off the heat and allow to cool for a few minutes until it is no longer steaming hot. Pour mixture into blender or Nutribullet for a smoother consistency (or mash by hand) with the butter or ghee and blend until smooth. At this time you might need to add more stock to keep it moving in the blender, and taste often for seasoning preferences. Scoop into a serving dish and enjoy!

Mashed Sweet Potatoes:

- Sweet potatoes (1/2 – 1 per person)
- Native Forest Unsweetened Coconut Milk (amount is not exact, add ¼ cup to start and add more if needed for preferred consistency)
- Celtic Sea Salt or Real salt and pepper to taste

Optional Add-Ins:

- 1 teaspoon of cinnamon
- 1 teaspoon nutmeg
- 1 teaspoon allspice
- 1 teaspoon freshly grated ginger

Directions:

1. Place peeled and cubed sweet potatoes in a pot of cold water on the stove.
2. Boil sweet potatoes until fork tender (about 10 minutes depending on how many you are making, the more you have in the pot, the longer they will take) then drain.
3. Add coconut milk, salt, pepper, and any optional add-ins you like and mash. Done!

Chocolate Pudding: (Please try this, I promise you will fall in love with it! It is so delicious you would never guess there is no dairy or sugar at all!)

- 2 ripe avocados
- ½ cup – 1 cup unsweetened vanilla coconut milk or nut/seed milk of choice (start with ½ cup and add more as you are blending to reach desired consistency)
- 1/8 – ¼ cup of unsweetened regular or dark cocoa powder (depending on level of chocolate intensity desired)
- Stevia to taste, I use about 3-4 teaspoons
- 1 teaspoon Frontier Vanilla extract (alcohol free)
- Pinch of Celtic Sea Salt

Directions:

1. Put all ingredients in a blender or Nutribullet and blend. You will have to shake it up and scrape down the sides a couple of times to make sure everything gets incorporated.
2. Add more unsweetened nut/seed milk of choice as needed to keep things blending and to reach desired consistency.

This recipe is also amazing because you can play around with it as much as you want as long as you use the base ingredients. You can add any flavors you want! In the fall I like to add a little pumpkin puree, cinnamon, and allspice for a chocolate pumpkin pudding, delicious! Or sometimes I add a tablespoon of instant coffee for a chocolate mocha pudding. Or just add some slivered almonds or chia seeds for a crunchy bite! The possibilities are only limited by your imagination and taste preferences.

Oven Baked Crispy Kale Chips:

- Kale leaves, enough to cover 1-2 baking sheets in a single layer (I buy it bagged and just tear out the ribs, but you can do the same for a head of kale, remove the ribs and chop it into chip-sized pieces)

- 2-4 tablespoons almond oil, avocado oil, or extra virgin olive oil
- Celtic Sea Salt or Real salt
- Any additional seasonings you like

Directions:

1. Set the oven to 275-280 and let it come all the way up to temperature before putting the kale in.
2. Thoroughly rinse and dry the kale leaves using a salad spinner or squeezing it tightly inside some paper or kitchen towels. **The drier it is, the crispier it will get.**
3. Line the baking sheets with aluminum foil and spread the kale out in a single layer. Drizzle oil over kale, enough to coat it but not enough to make any big pools of oil.
4. Sprinkle with the Celtic Sea Salt and other seasonings of choice, (make sure your hands are washed) and get in there and massage the oil and salt all over the kale coating each piece.
5. Make sure it is back in a single layer and put the kale in the oven. After 10 minutes take it out and turn the leaves over/move them around and put back in for 10 more minutes. Done! Warning: I usually eat 2 trays of it, it's so addictive!

Healthy Chicken Parmesan with Spaghetti Squash or Zucchini Noodles:

- Organic chicken breasts, chicken breast tenderloins, or boneless chicken thighs
- Jar of lowest sodium and lowest carb tomato sauce you can find, L.E. Roselli or Organicville for example OR make your own at home
- 1 spaghetti squash OR 1-2 organic zucchinis
- Organic mozzarella cheese
- Avocado or almond oil, or extra virgin olive oil
- Salt and pepper to taste
- Mrs. Dash Italian seasoning

Directions:

For Spaghetti Squash Option:

1. Set oven to 375.
2. Line a baking sheet with aluminum foil and lightly spray with non-stick cooking spray.
3. Cut spaghetti squash in half length-wise and scoop out the seeds.
4. Lightly drizzle the oil over the flesh of the squash and rub it in to make sure it covers the whole surface area.
5. Sprinkle with salt, pepper, and Italian seasoning, place them flesh side down on the baking sheet, and place in the oven for 45-50 minutes.
6. Remove the squash from the baking sheet and let cool for the time it takes to cook the chicken. When the chicken is done cooking, using a fork, scrape from top to bottom and remove the "spaghetti" from the squash into a serving bowl or plate.

For Zucchini Noodles Option:

7. I simply use a Veggetti Spiral Vegetable cutter that I got at my local supermarket. They also sell them at Walmart, Target, and on Amazon and other online retailers.
8. Place the "noodles" in a pan on low heat on the stove with a little bit of oil to coat them and a sprinkle of salt, pepper, and Italian seasoning
9. Let them get warm (about 5 minutes), then serve them with some sauce along-side the chicken.

For Chicken:

10. Place chicken on baking sheet lined with aluminum foil, sprinkle lightly with salt, pepper, and Italian seasoning, and put in oven for about 6 minutes for tenderloins or thin cut chicken breast. If it is thick cut, about 8 minutes.

11. After the first 6-8 minutes is up, take the chicken out, turn it over, first sprinkle about a tablespoon of cheese and then a tablespoon of sauce on top of the chicken.
12. Put chicken back in the oven for another 6-10 minutes until cooked through.

Quick Oven Baked Asparagus:

- Asparagus spears
- Salt and pepper to taste
- Garlic powder and onion powder (optional)
- Almond oil or extra virgin olive oil (cold pressed)

Directions:

1. Set oven to 400 and be sure to wait until it heats up to temperature before putting asparagus in.
2. Line a baking sheet with aluminum foil and spread asparagus out in a single layer.
3. Liberally coat asparagus with oil, then sprinkle with salt, pepper, garlic powder, and onion powder.
4. With clean hands, rub the oil and seasonings all over all of the asparagus and make sure they are back in a single layer.
5. Put them in the oven for 10-13 minutes depending on the strength of your oven or how you like your asparagus. The longer it's in, the crispier it will get.

Sweet Potato Brownies:

- 1 extra-large sweet potato (or 2-3 small), peeled and grated or baked and peeled
- 2 large eggs
- 1 tablespoon vanilla extract (Frontier, no alcohol)
- 3-4 tablespoons stevia (taste batter before baking to see if you want it sweeter)
- ½ cup   coconut oil, melted
- 1 tablespoon baking powder (reduced sodium and aluminum free if possible)

- ½ tablespoon baking soda
- 1 cup cocoa powder, unsweetened
- 2 tablespoons coconut flour

Directions:

1. Preheat oven to 365 Fahrenheit.
2. Combine the sweet potato, eggs, vanilla, and oil in a large bowl.
3. In a smaller bowl, combine the baking powder, baking soda, cocoa powder, stevia, and coconut flour and stir.
4. Stir the dry mixture into the wet mixture slowly until well combined.
5. Line an 8x8 cake pan with parchment paper. Spread the batter in the pan, and bake for 25-30 minutes.
6. Brownies are done when a toothpick inserted in the center comes out clean. Be careful not to over bake!
7. All the brownies to cool before removing from the pan. Enjoy, and be careful not to eat the whole tray in one sitting!

Amazing Protein Shake:

- 1 scoop protein powder of choice (I like Vega One Chocolate or Berry, or half a scoop of each!)
- 1 tablespoon Almond Butter or Peanut Butter
- 2 Ice Cubes
- 8-12 ounces of water or nut/seed milk of choice, or combo of water and nut/seed milk
- 2-4 Strawberries, frozen or fresh (optional)
- 1/8 teaspoon stevia (optional if you like it sweeter)

Directions:

Put all ingredients in a Nutribullet or blender and enjoy a delicious, sweet, guilt-free treat!

Oven Baked Sweet Potato Fries:

- 2-3 small sweet potatoes
- ¼ cup almond/avocado/melted coconut oil
- ½ tsp each salt, garlic, and onion powder
- ¼ tsp pepper
- Sprinkling of paprika

Directions:

1. Preheat oven to 425°, it is extremely important to make sure the oven has reached the temperature before you put the fries in.
2. Cut sweet potatoes into thin to medium cut fries (peeled or unpeeled, your choice) and place them in a large mixing bowl.
3. Add oil and all spices and mix with your hands until all the fries are evenly coated.
4. On a large sheet tray covered with parchment paper, spread the fries in one even layer and place them in the oven for 30 minutes, turning every 10 minutes with a spatula or just shake them around while wearing an oven mitt.
5. Keep an eye on them, because the thinner they are, the sooner they will be done/easier they will burn, and they may need to come out before 30 minutes is up.
6. Try to resist them for a minute when they are done and let them cool off so you don't burn your mouth, and enjoy!

Pumpkin Spiced Mixed Nuts and Seeds

- 1 egg white
- 1 teaspoon Celtic sea salt or Real salt
- 2 and ½ teaspoons allspice or pumpkin pie spice
- ¼ teaspoon cayenne pepper
- 3 teaspoons stevia
- 4 cups unsalted mixed nuts and seeds (my favorite combo is almonds, pecans, cashews, and pumpkin seeds)

Directions:

1. Preheat oven to 250 degrees Fahrenheit
2. Place egg white into a large bowl and whip with a fork until frothy
3. Stir in sea salt, spices and stevia
4. Combine mixture with 4 cups nuts/seeds and stir to coat them evenly
5. Place nuts/seeds in a single layer on top of a large parchment paper lined baking pan
6. Bake for 1 hour
7. Let nuts/seeds cool for at least 10 mins before serving (they will get crispy!)
8. Store in an airtight container for up to 2 weeks

ACKNOWLEDGMENTS

Since I aim to live in a state of gratitude, this section might end up longer than expected.

Firstly, thank you, Mom for always loving and nurturing me through all of the challenges we faced together, and never, ever letting me think that diabetes would limit what I could achieve in life. Thank you for instilling in me the love of traveling around the world and the love of cooking. And thank you for showing me the most shining example of what a strong, capable woman, who faces any and every obstacle that life throws at her with an open mind and a graceful heart, looks like so I could emulate it myself.

Thanks to my dad, who left us too soon, but not without many valuable life lessons. Thanks for having an entrepreneurial spirit, and for showing me that through hard work, you can realize your dreams. Thank you for showing me what true love looks like, and what I should expect in a husband by worshiping my mom like the goddess she is. And thank you for instilling in me one of the most important strengths to have in life…an unwavering sense of humor.

Thank you to my husband, Bill, who allowed me to discover what true love feels like, and to understand what the meaning of "soulmate" really is. Thank you for being my perfect partner in every aspect of life, and supporting every dream and aspiration I have, no matter how expansive it might be. Thank you for being the most intelligent, driven, loving, kind, generous, hard-working, inspirational man I have ever known. Thank you for having the indomitable strength to overcome your adversities so that those experiences could bring us together in that nightclub in Mexico where it all began. Thank you for calling me higher, and showing me that I always have just a little more left in me when I think I'm down for the count.

Thank you to my best friend, Alexis, for being there for me through every step of this journey we call life. For always having my back through every up and down. Thank you for all the laughter, for knowing what I'm thinking without having to say anything, and for speaking the language that only you and I can speak. For quite literally standing by my side through blood, sweat, and tears. Thank you for showing me what it truly means to have a sister.

Thank you to my favorite teacher of all time, Barry Fritz. If it weren't for your down to earth teaching style and kind encouragement, NPTI wouldn't have been nearly as much fun as it was. I actually looked forward to coming to school every day. And, you were the first person to teach me why my blood sugars spiked so high after lifting heavy! Thanks for all the valuable lessons.

Thank you to all of the incredibly inspiring people with diabetes who contributed their stories to this book, and for believing in my vision. Your bravery and willingness to openly share your stories and experiences has given me the courage to do the same. I am forever grateful for your support.

Thank you to the diabetes community. Thank you to every single person with diabetes. Thank you to every parent of a child with diabetes, every spouse, friend, and loved one of someone with diabetes who is there for us, and experiences the ups and downs with us. Without knowing that you are all out there and having the same day-to-day experiences that I am, I would have continued to feel alone like I did for so long. Knowing that my community of brothers and sisters are out there lets me feel like I am never alone. Thank you for being my fellow superheroes.

Thank you to all of my mentors in life who have taught me, and continue to teach me, the most valuable lessons in life, and inspire me to put no limits on what is possible: Tony and Sage Robbins, Napoleon Hill, Brendon Burchard, Les Brown, Bo and Dawn Eason, Dwayne "The Rock" Johnson, Brian Tracey, Oprah Winfrey, James Redfield, Wayne Dyer, Zig Ziglar, Jim Rohn, Bruce Lee, Nelson Mandela, Elon Musk, Stephen Colbert, Deepak Chopra, and Marianne Williamson. I am sure I'm not naming all of the incredible human beings, both living and past, who have inspired me to live with limitless passion and aspiration.

A very special thanks to Tony Robbins, whose teachings changed the course of my life entirely. It is because of your unbridled, unapologetic passion to help others understand what they are capable of that I found and embraced my personal power. It is because I consistently apply the lessons you teach that I am now living the life that I had previously only dreamed could be possible. I will forever be indebted to your deep love of service to humanity, and I will continually strive to pay your passions forward for as long as I live. I hear your voice in my own head every day, and for that I am forever grateful. Because of you: Now, I am the voice. I will lead, not follow. I will believe, not doubt. I will create, not destroy. I am a force for good. I am a leader. I will defy the odds. I will set a new standard. I will always STEP UP.

I could go on and on, but this is already a long book! I am eternally grateful.

CROWDFUNDING THANK YOU PAGE

These amazing people pledged to support our Kickstarter campaign at a significant level. Thank you for believing in our vision from the start!

Julie Jacky

Sherri Leigh Hollis

Jose and Carmen Gomez

Kathleen and Robert Starmer

James Stewart

Tom and Tara Hargenrader

Irene and Marc Lyman

Gayle Shapiro

Irene Sagalovsky

Bobbie Robertson

Judy Pousman

Book "Tweets" from Our High Level Pledgers:

Thank you for starting the much needed Diabetes Revolution, Daniele! You're an inspiration! <3 Love, Julie Jacky, Coach JulieJacky.com

You have my utmost love and respect Daniele! This is just the beginning for you. I see great things ahead for you because you have earned it through your hard work and dedication to diabetics around the world! YOU ROCK! –Sherri Leigh Hollis

"What you eat, you become" – Jose Gomez

ABOUT THE AUTHOR

Daniele Hargenrader, aka the Diabetes Dominator, is the bestselling author of *Unleash Your Inner Diabetes Dominator*. She is a nutritionist, diabetes and health coach, and certified personal trainer. She has been living with type 1 diabetes for almost 25 years, diagnosed in 1991. Daniele founded Diabetes Dominator in 2009 with the intention of serving those who are looking for a path to turn a perceived adversity into an advantage through the Diabetes Dominator system and the Six Pillars of Total Health. She helps individuals from all walks of life to think, eat, and move in ways that allow them to achieve a quality of health and life that they previously thought unattainable.

Daniele began her YouTube interview series, *Unleash Your Inner Diabetes Dominator,* in early 2015 in order to showcase as many positive role models in the diabetes community as possible. She wanted to clearly demonstrate that there are endless inspirational examples of the fact that living with diabetes should never be the reason we don't chase after our dreams and passions in life. Check out over 30 awesome interviews here: **youtube.com/824daniele**

She is an international speaker, has presented at Fortune 100 companies and top-ranked hospitals and universities, and has dedicated herself to teaching people how to live the life they imagined through optimal health. Daniele ballooned up to 200 pounds a few years after her diagnosis and the unexpected and sudden death of her father. She also battled depression and a binge eating addiction. Through these adversities, she eventually took herself from obese to athlete.

Daniele currently lives in Philadelphia (with an imminent move to southern California) with her husband, Bill, and their two cat children, Kitty and Frankie. Meet Daniele and receive free training and resources at **DiabetesDominator.com**.

23215870R00209

Made in the USA
Columbia, SC
05 August 2018